Praise for *Mastering Precepting: A Nurse's Handbook for Success*

"Mastering precepting is the only way the nursing profession will fulfill its promise to care as well as invest in its future—a future that ensures the next generation of nurses is safe, competent, and superbly qualified. The lessons and wisdom gained in *Mastering Precepting: A Nurse's Handbook for Success* will transform how you teach, learn, and become a professional nurse."

–Donna M. Nickitas, PhD, RN, NEA-BC, CNE
Hunter College, City University of New York Hunter-Bellevue School of Nursing
Deputy Executive Officer, Doctor of Nursing Science
Graduate Center, City University of New York
Editor, *Nursing Economic$*

"New preceptors need practical and pragmatic education and support as they move into this important role. *Mastering Precepting: A Nurse's Handbook for Success* explores precepting from all perspectives and provides practical advice to new preceptors as well as those who are experienced. Whether you are a new preceptor, a manager engaging preceptors in the onboarding of new staff, or a program director creating a preceptor program, *Mastering Precepting* will assist you in every phase of development. It is an excellent resource for a critical role."

–Kathleen A. Bower, DNSc, RN, FAAN
Principal and Co-owner, The Center for Case Management

"*Mastering Precepting: A Nurse's Handbook for Success* provides a timely pathway for preceptors to learn not only the intricacies of precepting, but also the responsibilities associated with this critical role. Dr. Ulrich articulates how to develop preceptors and, in turn, develop the nurses they precept. By recognizing precepting as a specialty that requires a unique set of knowledge and expertise, and providing a guide for organizations to ensure their preceptors are adequately prepared, *Mastering Precepting* contributes to developing the competent, engaged nurses who will be critical to the improvement of our nation's health care delivery organizations. What a great read!"

–Peter I. Buerhaus, PhD, RN, FAAN
Valere Potter Professor of Nursing
Director, Center for Interdisciplinary Health Workforce Studies
Institute for Medicine and Public Health
Vanderbilt University Medical Center

"Left to our own abilities, many of us would survive. But, why should we have such low expectations for what we could be as professional nurses? Creating the personal relationship that allows for coaching and openness will help us support learners in entry-level and advanced-role programs, new graduates in their transition into practice, and established practitioners in their transition from one role or clinical area to another. With the increasing focus on quality, safety, and competence in health care professions, we are fortunate to have strategies that support our ongoing development in these areas. Such is the case with *Mastering Precepting: A Nurse's Handbook for Success*."

–Patricia S. Yoder-Wise, EdD, RN, NEA-BC, ANEF, FAAN
President, The Wise Group

"The nursing preceptor role has taken on increasing significance in our complex health care environment. *Mastering Precepting: A Nurse's Handbook for Success* provides comprehensive, evidence-based, practical tools for precepting students in pre-licensure courses, newly-licensed nurses, experienced nurses moving from one institution or specialty to another, and internationally trained nurses."

–David R. Marshall, JD, DNP, RN, CENP, NEA-BC
Chief Nursing and Patient Care Services Officer
UTMB Health

"Now more than ever, we need to be successful in precepting the next generation of competent nurses to provide evidence-based care with compassion. *Mastering Precepting: A Nurse's Handbook for Success* brings us a well-researched collection of knowledge on how to best precept and also grounds the information in practical approaches to ensure success."

–Katherine Vestal, PhD, RN, FACHE, FAAN
President, Work Innovations LLC

"The practical principles and concepts and pragmatic tools shared throughout this book provide a framework for being an excellent team member as well as a preceptor. Ulrich and her contributing authors have been intentional with their content, using evidence as their foundation. Preceptors, preceptees, and managers will complete this book with a comprehensive new set of knowledge and a level of professional enthusiasm around making a difference in the lives of their colleagues."

–Rhonda Anderson, DNSc, RN, FAAN, FACHE
Chief Executive Officer, Cardon Children's Medical Center

"Effective precepting systems and processes are critical to enhancing new graduate competency skills and satisfaction with the work environment. In this new book, Beth Ulrich and contributors have captured the essence of the role as well as its value to the organization. Turnover rates continue to be high in the first year of employment for new RN graduates. The chapters address the multiple roles of preceptors that go beyond the traditional. Focusing on adult learning styles and available tools, as well as strategies for success, make this book a must for recruitment and retention."

–Roxane Spitzer, PHD, MBA, RN, FAAN
Editor-in-Chief, *Nurse Leader*

Mastering Precepting

A Nurse's Handbook for Success

Beth Tamplet Ulrich, EdD, RN, FACHE, FAAN

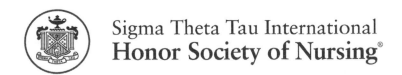

Sigma Theta Tau International
Honor Society of Nursing®

The Honor Society of Nursing, Sigma Theta Tau International (STTI) is a nonprofit organization whose mission is to support the learning, knowledge, and professional development of nurses committed to making a difference in health worldwide. Founded in 1922, STTI has 130,000 members in 86 countries. Members include practicing nurses, instructors, researchers, policymakers, entrepreneurs and others. STTI's 470 chapters are located at 586 institutions of higher education throughout Australia, Botswana, Brazil, Canada, Colombia, Ghana, Hong Kong, Japan, Kenya, Malawi, Mexico, the Netherlands, Pakistan, Singapore, South Africa, South Korea, Swaziland, Sweden, Taiwan, Tanzania, the United States, and Wales. More information about STTI can be found online at www.nursingsociety.org.

Sigma Theta Tau International
550 West North Street
Indianapolis, IN, USA 46202

To order additional books, buy in bulk, or order for corporate use, contact Nursing Knowledge International at 888.NKI.4YOU (888.654.4968/US and Canada) or +1.317.634.8171 (outside US and Canada).

To request a review copy for course adoption, e-mail solutions@nursingknowledge.org or call 888.NKI.4YOU (888.654.4968/US and Canada) or +1.317.917.4983 (outside US and Canada).

To request author information, or for speaker or other media requests, contact Rachael McLaughlin of the Honor Society of Nursing, Sigma Theta Tau International at 888.634.7575 (US and Canada) or +1.317.634.8171 (outside US and Canada).

ISBN-13:   978-1-935476-59-7
EPUB and Mobi ISBN: 978-1-935476-60-3
PDF ISBN: 978-1-935476-61-0

Library of Congress Cataloging-in-Publication Data

Mastering precepting: a nurse's handbook for success / [edited by] Beth Tamplet Ulrich.
    p. ; cm.
Includes bibliographical references.
ISBN 978-1-935476-59-7 (alk. paper)
1. Nursing--Study and teaching (Preceptorship) I. Ulrich, Beth Tamplet. II. Sigma Theta Tau International.
[DNLM: 1. Preceptorship. 2. Education, Nursing--methods. WY 18.5]
RT74.7.A78 2011
610.73--dc23
2011030044

Second Printing, 2015

Publisher: Renee Wilmeth   Principal Book Editor: Carla Hall
Acquisitions Editor: Cindy Saver   Project Editor: Katie Meyer-Cramer
Editorial Coordinator: Paula Jeffers   Copy Editor: Kevin Kent
Cover Designer: Michael Tanamachi   Proofreader: Jane Palmer
Indexer: Jane Palmer   Interior Design and Page Composition: Rebecca Batchelor

Dedication

To my husband, Walter, who is my biggest fan and supporter; to my daughter, Blythe, who makes me so proud to be her mom; and to my grandson, Henry, who brings me such joy.

To my colleagues who have precepted me throughout my career. I have been fortunate in every role I've ever held to have had someone who was willing to precept me—someone to help me transition to the new role and develop the competence and confidence to succeed. This book is dedicated to each of them with my utmost gratitude and appreciation.

To every nurse who has ever been a preceptor and every nurse who will become a preceptor. Your commitment to the nursing profession and to our patients makes me proud to be your colleague.

Acknowledgements

It truly takes a village to create a book.

Thank you first and foremost to a fantastic group of contributors. They are all preceptors themselves, and I appreciate their willingness to share their knowledge and expertise.

Thanks to my son-in-law, Michael McDonald, who created the book's website for preceptors (*www.RNPreceptor.com*) so that the work begun in the book can continue on and keep expanding.

Thanks to the wonderful Sigma Theta Tau International staff who takes care of every aspect of making a book idea come to life—with special thanks to Renee Wilmeth, who provided guidance, and Carla Hall, who provided encouragement and a sounding board.

About the Author

Beth Tamplet Ulrich, EdD, RN, FACHE, FAAN

Beth Ulrich is a nationally recognized thought leader who is known for her research studying nursing work environments and the experiences of new graduate nurses as they transition from nursing school into the workforce. She is also known for her leadership in developing the roles of nephrology nurses and improving the care of nephrology patients. Ulrich has extensive experience as a healthcare executive, educator, and researcher. She serves as senior partner at Innovative Health Resources, a company providing consultative services to health-care organizations and associations; as professor at the University of Texas Health Science Center at Houston School of Nursing; and as editor of Nephrology Nursing Journal, the professional journal of the American Nephrology Nurses' Association. Ulrich has been a co-investigator on a series of national nursing workforce and work environment studies, three studies of critical care nurse work environments conducted with the American Association of Critical-Care Nurses, and a national study on patient safety culture in nephrology nursing practice settings.

Ulrich received her bachelor's degree from the Medical University of South Carolina, her master's degree from the University of Texas Health Science Center at Houston, and her doctorate from the University of Houston in a collaborative program with Baylor College of Medicine. She is a past president of the American Nephrology Nurses' Association, a fellow in the American College of Healthcare Executives, and a fellow in the American Academy of Nursing. She was recognized as the Outstanding Nursing Alumnus of the Medical University of South Carolina in 1989 and as a Distinguished Alumnus of the University of Texas Health Science Center at Houston School of Nursing in 2002. She received the Outstanding Contribution to the American Nephrology Nurses' Association award in 2008. Ulrich is also a past member of the board of directors of the Foundation of the National Student Nurses' Association and recently served on the National Council of State Boards of Nursing Research Advisory Panel on Transition into Practice. She has numerous publications and presentations to her credit on nephrology nursing, nurses' work environments, transition of graduate nurses into professional nurses, and other topics.

Contributing Authors

Larissa Marquez Africa, MBA, BSN, RN

Larissa Africa is president of Versant. She began her nursing career at Children's Hospital Los Angeles (CHLA) as an RN resident and was involved in several unit-based activities, including precepting. Her involvement with the CHLA RN Residency expanded when she became curriculum coordinator, and soon after she became manager. Managing the RN Residency provided her with the opportunity to listen to preceptors and build tools to assist preceptors in their role. Africa's role in transitioning a department-based RN Residency to what is now Versant Holdings LLC has contributed to her knowledge of the pragmatics of precepting by learning from the best practice community of Versant clients.

Cherilyn Ashlock, MSN, RN

Cherilyn Ashlock has over 15 years of experience as a nurse specializing in pediatrics, RN transition to practice, and nursing excellence. In September 2013, Ashlock joined All Children's Hospital in St. Petersburg, Florida, to lead its Magnet designation efforts. Prior to her role at All Children's, she served as a national consultant with Versant RN Residency, assisting organizations across the country in the transition of newly graduated nurses to competent direct care providers. She has a passion for mentorship, leadership development, and professional nursing advancement.

Carol A. Bradley, MSN, RN, CENP

Carol Bradley is the senior vice president and system chief nursing officer for the Legacy Health System, a six-hospital integrated health care delivery system serving Portland, Oregon, and southwest Washington. Prior to joining Legacy, Bradley served in a variety of senior nursing executive positions in large health systems, including the not-for-profit, for-profit, and public hospital sectors, and was also the regional vice president and editor for the California edition of *NurseWeek*.

Within her nursing career, she has worked as a staff nurse, clinical specialist, clinical director, and senior nurse executive. Bradley holds associate and bachelor's degrees in nursing from the University of Nebraska and a Master of Science in Nursing degree from the University of Arizona. She is a 1991 Wharton Fellow and is certified in Executive Nursing

Practice (CENP) by the American Organization of Nurse Executives. She is a nationally known speaker and consultant on nursing/patient care, workforce issues, and work environment improvement, and is a frequent contributor to journals, media, and professional publications on topics important to nursing and patient care. She has contributed to several books and serves on the editorial board of *Nursing Administrative Quarterly.*

Thomas J. Doyle, MSN, RN

Tom Doyle has over 33 years experience in healthcare as a registered nurse, hospital administrator, nurse educator, and corporate executive. He is a recognized world expert in the use of experiential learning and simulation. Doyle spent five years as coordinator of the Patient Simulation Program at one of the first colleges in the United States to purchase the Human Patient Simulator in the 1990s, facilitating the integration of high fidelity patient simulation across the nursing program curriculum in addition to many allied health programs (EMS, dental hygiene, and respiratory care). He spent over 12 years as chief learning officer for METI/CAE Healthcare. In 2013, Doyle formed SimOne Healthcare Consultants LLC, which assists educators with applying, developing, implementing, and facilitating high fidelity simulation into their programs and also distributes e-Learning programs for healthcare. He is also a visiting fellow to the Faculty of Health, Science, and Sports at the University of South Wales in Pontypridd and a visiting research fellow to the Faculty of Health and Human Services at the University of Huddersfield, both in the United Kingdom.

Cathleen M. Deckers, EdD, RN

Cathy Deckers has over 15 years of nursing education and training experience in both the service and academic arenas. Her academic areas of expertise include utilization of high fidelity simulation for education training and competency assurance, management and supervision of clinical rotation experience, and data collection and research in clinical workforce. Deckers' research interests include the design of high fidelity simulation to develop expertise in decision-making. She currently is an assistant professor in the School of Nursing at California State University, Long Beach and also consults for CAE Healthcare, where she is responsible for successful implementation of simulation services related to nurse residency programs.

Amy K. Doepken, BSN, RN, CCRN

Amy Doepken is a registered nurse who works in the Kern Critical Care Unit at Legacy Good Samaritan Medical Center in Portland, Oregon. Her responsibilities include managing the unit training program, facilitating the debriefing program, running the clinical mentoring program, and functioning as a relief charge nurse. Doepken also works part-time for the Clinical Practice Department at Legacy Health, supporting the RN Residency program and the system-wide nurse precepting program for Legacy's six medical centers.

Doepken graduated with a Bachelor of Nursing Science from the University of Portland in 2002, received her CCRN certification in 2009, and is an active member of AACN. She began her career at Sacred Heart Medical Center in Eugene, Oregon, working in the Surgical and Trauma Critical Care Unit. In 2010, she was recognized for her precepting and mentoring work with a Legacy Health 2010 Circle of Excellence Award.

Denise D. Fall, BSN, RN

Denise Fall is the nurse manager of Legacy Health's Kern Critical Care Unit, which has received the Beacon Award for Critical Care Excellence. She joined the Kern Critical Care Unit in 2001 and worked as a staff nurse, preceptor, and charge nurse before assuming the role of nurse manager in 2007. Fall has successfully hired and transitioned new nurse graduates to her 28-bed, high-acuity critical care unit. Under her leadership, new nurse graduates are welcomed, supported, and mentored into her unit. She also believes in finding opportunities for her staff to be involved in nursing practice, whether on a unit or site, or on a system, local, or national level.

Fall received her Bachelor of Science in Nursing from Linfield College in Portland, Oregon, in 1998 and is currently pursuing her MSN in Healthcare Systems Management from Loyola University. She was the recipient of the Legacy Health 2010 Circle of Excellence Leadership Award and is a member of Sigma Theta Tau International, AACN, and AONE.

Mary Lyn Feldt, MSN, RN

Mary Lyn Feldt is a patient care specialist and RN Residency manager at Legacy Health. She received her master's in nursing care of children with a dual focus on clinical practice and nursing education from Case Western Reserve University. Feldt is experienced in clinical support, nursing education, and program development for acute care facilities, with more than 17 years of experience in supporting new employees (both experienced and new graduates) entering health care systems. She has developed and implemented multiple formal orientation programs, including formal preceptor and mentor programs, and has more than 14 years of experience as a children's clinical nurse specialist while building several growing pediatric service areas. She remains involved in clinical focus through the nurse residency. Feldt's focus is building and enhancing the onboarding and transition processes for nurses within Legacy Health via formal system-wide programs.

Mary S. Haras, PhD, MS, MBA, APN, NP-C, CNN

Mary Haras is associate dean for graduate nursing programs at Saint Xavier University School of Nursing in Chicago, Illinois. Haras has served as a preceptor and mentor to students, nurses, and faculty to acclimate them to their new roles. She is an adult nurse practitioner and is involved with the American Nephrology Nurses' Association with an interest in chronic kidney disease.

Cindy Lefton, PhD, RN

Cindy Lefton is manager and researcher, patient experience, emergency services at Barnes-Jewish Hospital and vice president of Organizational Consulting at Psychological Associates. She has combined her knowledge of organizations with her extensive experience as a registered nurse, paramedic, and clinical research nurse to develop a variety of effective interventions for academic medical centers and hospitals. These projects encompass a broad scope of services, including coaching, team building, survey development, and organizational collaboration training. Her research interests include healthy work environments, demonstrating respect in the workplace, and collaboration between nurses and ancillary services partners. Lefton leads The DAISY Award Impact Research team. She has published articles on collaboration, respect, and culture change and led the AONE, ARAMARK, and Studer Group research team to develop and validate the NS3, a survey that assesses nurse satisfaction with support services. She continues to practice as an emergency department RN at Saint Mary's Health Center in St. Louis.

Lefton obtained her PhD in psychology from St. Louis University. She earned a Master of Science Research from St. Louis University and a Master of Arts in human resource management from Washington University, a Bachelor of Science in industrial psychology and organizational psychology from Washington University, and a nursing diploma from Jewish Hospital School of Nursing.

Karen C. Robbins, MS, RN, CNN

Karen Robbins is the independent living donor advocate in collaboration with the Hartford Transplant Program at Hartford Hospital in Hartford, Connecticut. She is associate editor of *Nephrology Nursing Journal,* the official journal of the American Nephrology Nurses' Association, and a past national president of the American Nephrology Nurses' Association. She has been a nurse educator for dialysis and transplant programs; a nurse clinician in transplantation; a mentor and educator for many nurses, particularly in nephrology nursing; and a clinical faculty member. She is a published author, editor, experienced speaker, and legal nurse consultant. Most recently, she served as co-editor of the second edition of *Applying Continuous Quality Improvement in Clinical Practice.*

Kim A. Richards, RN

As a nurse and an executive recruiter, Kim Richards became increasingly aware of the "revolving door" of nurses in acute care facilities. After interviewing hundreds of nurses, she noticed a common theme was emerging. Nurses were expressing signs and symptoms of compassion fatigue, a debilitating phenomenon that is caused by years of built-up emotional residue. By combining her passion for nursing, fitness, and coaching with her extensive research on the science of self-care, Richards created the components of Self-Care Academy, LLC, a comprehensive program that is dedicated to improving employee engagement and relationships with peers and to creating an optimum healing environment for patients. An author, professional speaker, and health coach, Richards is passionate about supporting busy caregivers in their quest for practical self-care integration.

Laurie Shiparski, MS, BSN, RN

Laurie Shiparski has more than 30 years of experience in nursing and health care leadership positions. She has worked in various roles, including critical care RN, clinical hospital leadership, health care consulting business owner, and corporate executive in a health care technology and clinical practice company. She is a senior vice president at Verras Consulting. Her focus in consulting has included leadership development and coaching, interdisciplinary communication and partnership, physician-driven practice improvement, creating healthy work cultures, and advancing evidence-based practice and technology to improve interdisciplinary care.

Shiparski has sought to uncover her gifts and bring her authentic self to work and life, which has inspired her to offer programs that focus on taking care of self, navigating change, finding passion and purpose, and creating new possibilities. She is also an international speaker and an author of numerous articles and five books.

Jennifer L. Thornburgh, BSN, RN

Jennifer Thornburgh is an emergency department nurse manager with Legacy Health in Portland, Oregon. She has more than 17 years experience in emergency nursing and has worked in various roles, including staff RN, preceptor, nurse educator, charge nurse, legal nurse consultant, emergency management coordinator, nursing supervisor, and manager.

Thornburgh believes that new graduate nurses can be successful in the emergency department, and their success is highly dependent on both a robust didactic experience and a strong preceptor support program. In her role as manager, she co-chairs the Preceptor Development and Support Committee at Legacy Health. This group refined Legacy's preceptor program with a focus on objective preceptor selection criteria, preceptor education, and ongoing support of the preceptor.

Wendy Jo Wilkinson, MSN, ARNP

Wendy Jo Wilkinson has more than 35 years of experience in the health care industry, serving in various roles within the acute hospital setting, home health care operations, and education. In these roles, she has gained expertise in leadership, multisite management, start-up operations, strategic and financial planning, establishing clinical standards and competencies, development of specialized clinical programs, quality management and improvement, customer relations, and sales and marketing initiatives. Wilkinson now serves as director of academic and hospital services for CAE Healthcare, managing a team that consults and assists customers with applying, developing, implementing, and facilitating high fidelity patient simulation into their academic and hospital-based programs, and is ultimately responsible for oversight of all of CAE Healthcare's learning products to ensure they are clinically and pedagogically sound.

Collista J. Zook, MS, CNS, RN

Collista Zook is the clinical nurse specialist (CNS) for emergency and trauma services at Legacy Health in Portland, Oregon, and Vancouver, Washington. Before joining Legacy, she was the CNS for emergency services at a central Oregon hospital and a CNS/educator for the critical care department of a hospital in central Kansas. Zook graduated with a Diploma in Nursing from Baptist Hospital School of Nursing in St. Louis, Missouri, and received her Bachelor of Science in Nursing and Master of Science in Nursing degrees from Kansas University Medical Center in Kansas City, Kansas. In 2001, she completed her postgraduate education and certification in forensic nursing (concentration in injury and death investigation) from Beth-El College of Nursing & Health Sciences, University of Colorado at Colorado Springs, Colorado.

Zook has 35 years in nursing, using her nursing knowledge and skills in a variety of clinical, public health, and specialty areas of nursing practice. She has also been a guest lecturer for trauma symposiums and key speaker for nursing and state investigators in forensic recognition and documentation. She sits on the Oregon State Board of Nursing's Nurse Practice Council. Zook has developed, redesigned, and assisted in implementation of preceptor programs in many of the facilities she has been employed with and continues to support the embracing of ideals and freshness that accompany "new grads" in their first career positions as "new nurses."

Table of Contents

Introduction xxi

1 The Preceptor Role 1

Beth Tamplet Ulrich

The Context of Precepting 2

Preceptor Roles 8

   Teacher/Coach 8

   Leader/Influencer 9

   Facilitator 10

   Evaluator 11

   Socialization Agent 12

   Protector 12

   Role Model 13

Conclusion 13

   References 13

2 Learning: The Foundation of Precepting 17

Beth Tamplet Ulrich

Adult Learning Theory 17

Transformative Learning Theory 20

Social Learning Theory 20

Hierarchy of Needs Theory 21

From Novice to Expert 23

Learning Styles 25

Curry's Learning Style Classification System 26

Cognitive Styles 26

   Gregorc's Learning Styles 26

   Myers-Briggs 27

   Field Dependence/Independence 28

Information Processing Styles 28

Instructional Preferences 30

Sensory Learning Styles 30

Conclusion: Preceptor as Learner and Preceptor as Teacher 30

   References 31

3 Precepting Strategies 35

Beth Tamplet Ulrich

Getting Started 35

Precepting Models 37

Single Preceptor Model *37*
Team Preceptor Model *37*
Preceptee Cohorts or One at a Time? 38
Sharing Information 39
It Takes a Village 40
Establishing the Preceptor-Preceptee Relationship 41
Preceptee Learner Assessment 42
Managing Transitions 42
Clinical Teaching Strategies 43
Strengths-Based Approach *43*
Microskills Model *45*
Debriefing *47*
Reflective Practice *49*
Ending the Preceptor-Preceptee Relationship 49
Conclusion 50
References *51*

**4   Competence, Critical Thinking, Clinical Judgment and
Reasoning, and Confidence** **55**
Beth Tamplet Ulrich

Competence 55
Conscious Competence Learning *57*
Competency Outcomes and Performance Assessment (COPA) Model *57*
Competence Development *58*
Critical Thinking 59
Critical Thinking—A Philosophical Perspective *60*
Critical Thinking in Nursing *62*
Precepting Critical Thinking *63*
Clinical Reasoning 64
Clinical Judgment 65
Developing Expert Reasoning and Intuition 67
Confidence 69
Conclusion 69
References *70*

**5   Having a Plan: Developing and Using Objectives,
Goals, and Outcomes** **75**
Karen C. Robbins and Mary S. Haras

Expectations 76
The Relationship Among Goals, Objectives, and Outcomes 77
Objectives vs. Outcomes *77*

Learning Taxonomies.. 79

Bloom's Taxonomy: Objectives and Domains of Learning.......................*79*

Fink's Taxonomy of Significant Learning *87*

Behavioral Objectives 90

Creating Outcome Statements 91

Distinguishing Outcomes From Objectives 92

Developing Measurable Objectives and Outcomes..................... 93

Pitfalls of Developing Objectives *95*

Conclusion 97

References *97*

6 Communication.. 103

Laurie Shiparski

The Five Skills of Effective Communication........................... 103

Intent 105

Listening 106

Advocacy 108

Inquiry... 110

Silence 112

Managing Different Methods of Communication...................... 112

Patient Safety and Handoffs 112

Considerations for Participating in Team Communications............ 114

Managing Difficult Conversations 115

Strategies for Education and Meetings 116

Conclusion 118

References 118

Additional Resources 119

7 Coaching 121

Laurie Shiparski

What Is the Role of the Preceptor as Coach?........................... 121

Setting Up a Coaching Agreement With a Preceptee 122

Utilizing a Coaching Interaction Format 123

Strategies to Inspire Learning and Move Through Challenges.......... 129

The Preceptor's Role in Working With Resistance and Edges........... 130

An Edge Story 131

Ending a Coaching Relationship With a Preceptee..................... 132

Conclusion 133

References 133

Additional Resources 133

8 Effectively Using Instructional Technologies 135
Cathleen M. Deckers, Thomas J. Doyle, Wendy Jo Wilkinson

E-Learning 135
Web-Based Collaboration Tools 137
    Effectiveness of Web-Based Collaboration Tools 138
Simulation 139
    The Pursuit of Fidelity 139
High-Fidelity Patient Simulation 142
    Developing Clinical Competence and Confidence 143
    Facilitating Clinical Judgment 143
    Developing Situation Awareness and Clinical Reasoning 144
    Design of High-Fidelity Patient Simulation Experiences 145
    Implications of Using High-Fidelity Patient Simulation for Preceptors,
    Educators, and Managers 148
    Quality Improvement 152
New Learners—The Net Generation 153
Future of Instructional Technology/Future Implications of
Instructional Technology Use 154
    References 155

9 Precepting Specific Learner Populations 159
Beth Tamplet Ulrich

Pre-Licensure Student Nurses 159
    Creating a Positive Clinical Learning Environment 163
    A Recruitment Strategy 164
New Graduate Nurses 164
    The Practice-Education Gap 165
    Bridging the Gap—Transition to Practice 165
    Precepting New Graduate Nurses 166
    Managing the Normal Chaos 167
    Scope of Practice and Autonomy 167
    Other Considerations With New Graduates 168
Experienced Nurses 169
Internationally Educated Nurses 170
Nurses From Different Generations 171
    Learning Styles and Preferences 173
    Precepting and Working With Each Generation 173
Conclusion 173
    References 174

10   Assessing and Addressing Preceptee Behavior and Motivation . . . 177
Cindy Lefton

Just Culture: A Problem-Solving Framework 179
   Three Types of Errors. 179
   Applying Just Culture 180
Providing Feedback 182
The Dimensional Model of Behavior 182
Motivation. 188
Interacting with Influence—The Five Step Format. 190
   Step One: Start the Conversation 191
   Step Two: Get the Preceptee's Views 192
   Step Three: Give Your Views (of the Preceptee's Views) 193
   Step Four: Resolve Differences 194
   Step Five: Developing an Action Plan 194
Conclusion 195
   References 196

11   Pragmatics of Precepting. 199
Larissa Marquez Africa and Cherilyn Ashlock

Organization and Time Management. 199
   Preparing for the Shift and Patient Assignment 200
   Shift Report 200
   The Preceptor and Preceptee Shift 200
   Establishing a Routine and Facilitating Prioritization. 201
Delegation. 203
Performance Discrepancies 206
Problem Solving Preceptor-Preceptee Relationships. 208
   When Skill Development Becomes a Challenge 208
Challenging Behaviors 210
   Preceptor-Preceptee Mismatch. 210
Conclusion 211
   References 211

**12   For Managers: Selecting, Supporting, and
     Sustaining Preceptors 213**
*Carol A. Bradley, Amy K. Doepken, Denise D. Fall, Mary L. Feldt,
Jennifer L. Thornburgh, and Collista J. Zook*

Establishing Performance Standards 214
Developing the Foundation—Preceptor Selection Criteria 216
Setting the Stage. 220
Conflict Considerations. 221
Preceptor Education. 222

Communication. 223
Guidance 224
Preceptor Evaluation 225
Recognition of Preceptors 227
Getting Creative to Overcome Challenges 229
Conclusion 230
  References *230*

**13 The Practice of Self-Care to Prevent Burnout and
    Create the Optimal Healing Environment. 233**
Kim Richards

Physical. 234
Mental. 235
Emotional 237
Spiritual 239
Relationships 239
Choices. 240
Conclusion 242
  References *242*

Appendix **245**

Index. **255**

Foreword *by Kathy Sanford*

Sometimes when I'm reminiscing with colleagues of my generation, we engage in discussions about our early days in acute care practice. Invariably, many of us describe our first hospital caregiver experiences as less than smooth. We ruefully speak of our personal lack of organization skills, early patient care errors, inadequate coping abilities, culture shock, and—most of all—our fear. We share that we were afraid of looking foolish; afraid of not knowing how to respond to disrespectful treatment from other clinicians; and, foremost in our minds, afraid of causing harm to our patients.

The most common description of our orientation to the life of a clinical nurse is that we were "thrown into the role" with inadequate understanding of, or preparation for, our responsibilities. We shake our heads and wonder how our patients survived our lack of expertise, and how *we* survived and thrived in this gloriously complex profession. Then we remember that some of our past friends and coworkers have not shared in this long-term experience. They chose not to stay in the field. We've all met people who introduce themselves as someone who "used to be a nurse." As I read my advance copy of this handbook, I theorized about how many of these former clinicians might still be contributing their talents and education to patient care if their early experiences had included the guidance and coaching of their more experienced peers.

Today, we try to do a better job of onboarding new nursing team members. Almost every organization has some sort of organized orientation program. Many have formally designated preceptor programs. In spite of these improvements, turnover among new graduates remains high. Some early-career nurses describe their first year in the workforce in much the same way as my contemporaries do. We are still on the journey toward finding a way to provide a better transition from student to graduate nurse. *Mastering Precepting: A Nurse's Handbook for Success* is a tool to help us get there. It focuses on improving the skills of those who serve as preceptors, not only for new graduates but for nurses transitioning from any nursing role into another. Its underlying premise is that we can improve our precepting abilities and, in doing so, can contribute to the enrichment of other nurses' careers.

It's rewarding to think that each of us can have a positive influence on one individual's professional life, but the one-to-one relationship that a preceptor and preceptee develop is not the sum total of what excellent precepting can do for our organizations, our communities, and our profession. How many nurses will become more skilled at what they do because of programs designed to support students, new graduates, new hires, and colleagues who are moving into a new specialty? How many might extend their nursing careers as a result? How many patients will receive safe, quality care because of a well-crafted precepting program?

There is a correlation among these questions, of course. Individuals who continue to practice nursing mitigate community shortages of caregivers. Communities and patients receive better care from competent, self-assured, and assertive nurses. Preceptors help their less experienced colleagues gain this competency, self-assurance, and assertiveness. That is, they serve as guides for this professional development—but only if they themselves are skilled in the art and science of precepting.

Beth Ulrich and the contributing authors of this book clearly understand that there is more to serving as a preceptor than a title or having enough experience in a job to orient a new team member to policies, procedures, and "the way we do things around here." Their attention to this role indicates a deep respect for the skilled nurse preceptor, an appreciation for the responsibility and challenges involved in the work of competent precepting, and a recognition of the far-reaching influence preceptors have on nursing careers and patient care. Chapter by chapter, these experts share their experience, dispensing useful advice along with enough underlying theory and research findings to explain why the practical applications work. The "handbook" title is accurate: This collection of topics adds up to a volume that can serve not only as a primer for a new preceptor but a resource to consult as needed over a lifetime of precepting.

It's clear that the authors hope that readers who choose to be preceptors will continue to perform in this role throughout their careers. They understand that the proficiencies of a good nurse preceptor, like the proficiencies of a good nursing manager, are not inherent in everyone. Even those who are predisposed to mentor or aid others in their career development need to learn and practice new skills. There are competencies that are separate from other clinical abilities that make the preceptor's role a specialty or, if you prefer, a subspecialty to a major clinical specialty.

This book is a gift to nursing, not just to those who choose to serve as a preceptor. If you read it from start to finish, you will have a thorough picture of the role. You will have a better understanding of how important each precepting opportunity is to the future of nursing and health care. Finally, you'll have practical steps to take as you serve as guide and coach to an individual professional colleague.

–Kathy Sanford, DBA, RN, CENP, FACHE
Sr. Vice President/Chief Nursing Officer
Catholic Health Initiatives

Foreword *by Gwen Sherwood*

There are many approaches to teaching and learning; learning "by doing" is a time-honored pedagogy for service professions. Indeed, the apprentice style is a major point of discussion in the 2010 book *Educating Nurses: A Call for Radical Transformation* (Benner, Sutphen, Leonard, & Day). Learning by doing is not haphazard trial and error, but requires systematic approaches based on learner objectives negotiated between preceptee and preceptor, consideration of learning styles and learning context, and effective use of available resources. To learn by doing involves careful coaching, facilitation, mentoring, guidance, and supervision by a skilled practitioner of the craft being learned. While supervision from preceptors is a standard learning approach, our profession has often overlooked the special skills required of excellent preceptors, and the point that not all great clinicians make effective preceptors. Good precepting, like good teaching or good nursing care, is a carefully developed expertise that evolves over time. *Mastering Precepting: A Nurse's Handbook for Success* fills the gap by offering a comprehensive guide to the apprenticeship learning model for nurse educators, managers, and preceptors.

Teaching involves craft. There is both an art and a science in teaching preceptors as well. Preceptors not only guide skill acquisition based on the science of nursing—they also practice the art of nursing by helping learners reflect on their experiences to examine the meaning, objectively looking at varying perspectives of an event, to "make sense" of it within the context of empirical knowledge as well as other circumstances that influence the situation. Reflecting-in and reflecting-on action to learn from one's experiences are the bases of Benner's (1984) *From Novice to Expert*. Preceptors are front-line guides who observe the learner's developing competencies and thus have a key role in evaluation and assessment.

At all levels and in all settings, the work of nursing is physically and emotionally intense. A lack of opportunity to reflect on practice to make sense of events can lead to burnout; the complexities of relationships and caregiving need to be examined in a systematic way and wrestled with to come to terms with how to balance the ideal response with the reality of the course of events to reach a resolution for changing the response in future situations. For most learners, this requires a guide, coach, facilitator, or mentor who can enter the dialogue and offer alternative perspectives and assessment.

Authored by an experienced educator, scholar, and clinician who has been closely involved in developing transition to practice programs for new graduate nurses, this book provides clear steps for preceptor orientation, qualifications, and skills to prepare preceptors for their key role in education. Reflective teachers themselves must be able to reflect to make sense of their teaching. *Mastering Precepting* does not leave preceptor preparation to chance, but offers a toolkit to effective competency development. It is a book that all nursing education programs should have, whether located in clinical settings for transition to practice programs and new employee orientation, or in academic settings for guiding learners in a capstone course or advanced practice clinical experiences.

Preceptors support the pillars of education by guiding preceptees in learning to do, know, be, and work/live together. As key role models, they are in a sense the keepers of our discipline by linking the learner's education foundation with the clinical world. They themselves must understand the double helix of the theoretical basis for nursing practice, and how that feeds back into educational development in seeking knowledge to have relevant evidence for care delivery. This critical book helps recognize the art and the science of excellent precepting, helping learners bridge the nursing education and practice worlds.

–Gwen Sherwood, PhD, RN, FAAN
Professor and Associate Dean for Academic Affairs
University of North Carolina at Chapel Hill School of Nursing
Co-Investigator, QSEN (Quality and Safety Education for Nurses)

References

Benner, P. (1984). From novice to expert: Excellence and power in clinical nursing practice. Menlo Park, CA: Addison-Wesley Publishing.

Benner, P., Sutphen, M., Leonard, V., & Day, L. (2010). Educating nurses: A call for radical transformation. San Francisco, CA: Jossey-Bass.

Introduction

"Live as if you were going to die tomorrow.
Learn as if you were going to live forever."
–Mahatma Gandhi

Preceptors live at the intersections of education and practice and of the present and the future. They practice at the point where theoretical learning meets reality and where the gap between current and needed knowledge and expertise gets filled. Preceptors are the essential link between what nurses are taught and what they do, and between what nurses know and what they need to know. Having competent preceptors is critical to educating nursing students, transitioning new graduate nurses to the professional nursing role, and transitioning experienced nurses to new roles and specialties.

Preceptors teach at the point of practice. They create experiences in which the preceptee can engage and learn. Benner and colleagues (2010, p. 42) note that "only experiential learning can yield the complex, open-ended, skilled knowledge required for learning to recognize the nature of the particular resources and constraints in equally open-ended and undetermined clinical situations," and that "experiential learning depends on an environment where feedback in performance is rich and the opportunities for articulating and reflecting on the experiences are deliberately planned" (p. 43). Teaching/precepting is a two-way street—it requires a constant back-and-forth communication between the preceptor and the preceptee. Preceptors use listening and observation skills as much or more than talking and doing skills.

Myths

Several myths about preceptors and precepting need to be dispelled. The first is that because you are a good clinical nurse, you will be a good preceptor. While preceptors do indeed need to be competent in the area of nursing they will be precepting, becoming a preceptor is like learning a new clinical specialty. While some previously learned knowledge and skills are useful, there are many more to be learned before you become a competent preceptor. The next myth is that you have to be an expert clinician to be a preceptor. In many cases, being much more expert than the person you are precepting can be a hindrance and is frustrating to the preceptor and the preceptee. Yet another myth is that precepting must work around whatever patient assignment is made and whatever is happening on the unit. Such activity is not precepting. It is ineffective at its best and, at its worse, disheartening and anxiety-provoking for the preceptor and the preceptee. Every nurse deserves a competent preceptor and a safe, structured environment in which to learn. That is not to say that every precepting activity will go as planned. It will not. There is much unpredictability in the nursing work environment, but precepting activities must start with a plan based on the needs of the preceptee and the outcomes that must be obtained. Part of the competence of preceptors is making the plan, adjusting when the need arises, and recognizing and using teachable moments.

Who Should Read This Book

This book is a survival guide for preceptors and precepting. It is a resource for preceptors from two perspectives—the knowledge they need to become competent preceptors and the knowledge they need to precept others.

The book is both evidence-based and pragmatic. It provides information on the why and the how, and is written in a style that can be easily read by busy staff nurses who are moving into the preceptor role and by current preceptors who want to improve their practice. The information in the book can be immediately integrated into practice. The book can also serve as a resource for preceptor education programs.

Book Content

The chapters in the book build on each other and are designed to be read in order. Chapter 1 is an introduction to precepting and discusses all the aspects of the preceptor role. Chapter 2 discusses how individuals learn. Chapter 3 offers an overview of precepting strategies, beginning with the preceptor and manager setting role expectations and responsibilities. Chapter 4 is about planning the preceptee's experiences and developing and using objectives, goals, and outcomes. Chapter 6 discusses communication skills. Chapter 7 provides information on coaching. Chapter 8 presents an overview of instructional technologies— from web-based strategies to human patient simulation—and details on when and how to use the technologies effectively. Chapter 9 offers information and strategies on specific learner populations—new graduate nurses, experienced nurses learning new specialties or roles, internationally educated nurses, and nurses from different generations. Chapter 10 has details on assessing and addressing preceptee behaviors and motivation. Chapter 11 offers pragmatic information on the day-to-day performance of the precepting role. Chapter 12 is designed for managers and discusses how to select, support, and sustain preceptors. Chapter 13 discusses the need for preceptors to practice self-care behaviors and provides suggestions to prevent burnout and create optimal healing environments. The Appendix contains suggestions for using each chapter in preceptor education programs.

At the end of each chapter, you will find a Preceptor Development Plan. The first part of the plan is a set of questions to reflect on after reading the chapter. These questions help you think about your own strengths and needs. The second part of the Preceptor Development Plan is a template for you to use to create your own plan. The templates are available on our website (*www.RNPreceptor.com*) as modifiable documents and can be used by individuals or by organizations. By putting your own plan in writing, you will be making a commitment to implement the plan. For organizations, the plans can be used to set goals and measure progress for participants in preceptor education programs.

More Information Online

To accompany this book, we have also created a website—*www.RNPreceptor.com*—which provides additional resources for preceptors and preceptor training. It also has a message board for preceptors to communicate with each other and to share problems and solutions.

Final Thoughts

Precepting is a complex endeavor that requires competence and commitment. By becoming a preceptor, you have accepted the professional responsibility of sharing your knowledge and expertise with others. There is no greater contribution to nursing and to patient care than to ensure the competence of the next generation of nurses.

You raise me up so I can stand on mountains
You raise me up to walk on stormy seas
I am strong when I am on your shoulders
You raise me up to more than I can be
(Lovland & Graham, 2003)

–Beth Tamplet Ulrich, EdD, RN, FACHE, FAAN
BethUlrich@aol.com

References

Benner, P., Sutphen, M., Leonard, V., & Day, L. (2010). *Educating nurses: A call for radical transformation.* San Francisco, CA: Jossey-Bass.

Lovland, R., & Graham, B. (2003). You raise me up. [Recorded by Josh Groban]. On Closer [CD]. Burbank, CA: Reprise Records.

"No one was ever able to teach who was not able to learn."

–Florence Nightingale

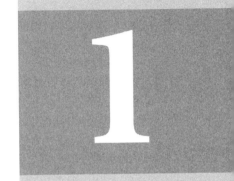

The Preceptor Role

Beth Tamplet Ulrich, EdD, RN, FACHE, FAAN

Precepting is an organized, evidence-based, outcome-driven approach to assuring competent practice. Precepting is used for students who are rotating into clinical areas, for new graduate nurse onboarding, for new hire onboarding, when experienced staff members learn a new specialty or new skills, and when individuals move into new roles (i.e., educator, manager, or preceptor). A preceptor is an individual with demonstrated competence in a specific area who serves as a teacher/coach, leader/influencer, facilitator, evaluator, socialization agent, protector, and role model to develop and validate the competencies of another individual. This chapter presents an overview of precepting and the preceptor role.

Precepting takes place in the context of the health care system and involves many role functions. A precepting model that illustrates the roles and context of precepting is shown in Figure 1.1.

OBJECTIVES

- Understand precepting in the context of nursing and the health care system

- Understand the role of a preceptor

- Know the competencies required to practice as a preceptor

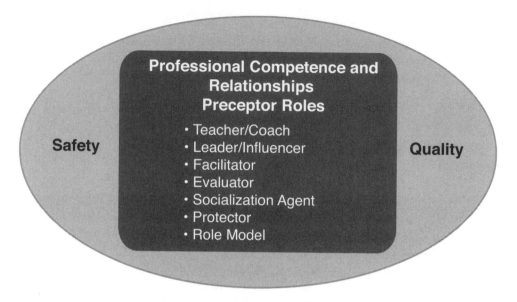

Figure 1.1   Precepting Model

The Context of Precepting

Precepting takes place in nursing and in the broader health care system. Professional nursing practice is complex and multifaceted. At its most basic, nursing is defined as "the protection, promotion, and optimization of health and abilities, prevention of illness and injury, alleviation of suffering through the diagnosis and treatment of human response and advocacy in the care of individuals, families, communities, and populations" (American Nurses Association [ANA], 2010a, p. 3).

Nursing has evolved into a profession that has a distinct body of knowledge, a social contract, and an ethical code. Nursing standards of practice describe a competent level of nursing care, and standards of professional performance describe a competent level of behavior in the professional role (ANA, 2010b; see Table 1.1). In addition, the ANA Code of Ethics for Nurses provides a succinct statement of the ethical obligations and duties of every nurse. This code is the profession's nonnegotiable ethical standard and is an expression of nursing's own understanding of its commitment to society (ANA, 2001; see Table 1.2). Preceptors need to be grounded in these standards.

Table 1.1   Standards of Nursing Practice (ANA, 2010b, pp. 9-11)

Standards of Practice

Standard 1. Assessment. The registered nurse collects comprehensive data pertinent to the health care consumer's health and/or the situation.

Standard 2. Diagnosis. The registered nurse analyzes the assessment data to determine the diagnoses or issues.

Standard 3. Outcomes Identification. The registered nurse identifies expected outcomes for a plan individualized to the health care consumer or the situation.

Standard 4. Planning. The registered nurse develops a plan that prescribes strategies and alternatives to attain expected outcomes.

Standard 5. Implementation. The registered nurse implements the identified plan.

>   **Standard 5A. Coordination of Care.** The registered nurse coordinates care delivery.

>   **Standard 5B. Health Teaching and Health Promotion.** The registered nurse employs strategies to promote health and a safe environment.

>   **Standard 5C. Consultation.** The graduate level-prepared specialty nurse or advanced practice registered nurse provides consultation to influence the identified plan, enhance the abilities of others, and effect change.

>   **Standard 5D. Prescriptive Authority and Treatment.** The advanced practice registered nurse uses prescriptive authority, procedures, referrals, treatments, and therapies in accordance with state and federal laws and regulations.

Standard 6. Evaluation. The registered nurse evaluates progress towards the attainment of outcomes.

Standards of Professional Performance

Standard 7. Ethics. The registered nurse practices ethically.

Standard 8. Education. The registered nurse attains knowledge and competence that reflects current nursing practice.

Standard 9. Evidence-based Practice and Research. The registered nurse integrates evidence and research findings into practice.

Standard 10. Quality of Practice. The registered nurse contributes to quality nursing practice.

Standard 11. Communication. The registered nurse communicates effectively in all areas of practice.

Standard 12. Leadership. The registered nurse demonstrates leadership in the professional practice setting and the profession.

Standard 13. Collaboration. The registered nurse collaborates with the health care consumer, family, and others in the conduct of nursing practice.

Standard 14. Professional Practice Evaluation. The registered nurse evaluates his or her own nursing practice in relation to professional practice standards and guidelines, relevant statutes, rules, and regulations.

Table 1.1   Standards of Nursing Practice (ANA, 2010b, pp. 9-11) (cont.)

Standard 15. Resource Utilization. The registered nurse utilizes appropriate resources to plan and provide nursing services that are safe, effective, and financially responsible.

Standard 16. Environmental Health. The registered nurse practices in an environmentally safe and healthy manner.

Table 1.2   ANA Code of Ethics (ANA, 2001)

Provision 1. The nurse, in all professional relationships, practices with compassion and respect for the inherent dignity, worth, and uniqueness of every individual, unrestricted by considerations of social or economic status, personal attributes, or the nature of health problems.

Provision 2. The nurse's primary commitment is to the patient, whether an individual, family, group, or community.

Provision 3. The nurse promotes, advocates for, and strives to protect the health, safety, and rights of the patient.

Provision 4. The nurse is responsible and accountable for individual nursing practice and determines the appropriate delegation of tasks consistent with the nurse's obligation to promote optimum patient care.

Provision 5. The nurse owes the same duties to self as to others, including the responsibility to preserve integrity and safety, to maintain competence, and to continue personal and professional growth.

Provision 6. The nurse participates in establishing, maintaining, and improving health care environments and conditions of employment conducive to the provision of quality health care and consistent with the values of the profession through individual and collective action.

Provision 7. The nurse participates in the advancement of the profession through contributions to practice, education, administration, and knowledge development.

Provision 8. The nurse collaborates with other health professionals and the public in promoting community, national, and international efforts to meet health care needs.

Provision 9. The profession of nursing, as represented by associations and their members, is responsible for articulating nursing values, for maintaining the integrity of the profession and its practice, and for shaping social policy.

Over the past decade, the Institute of Medicine (IOM) and other agencies and associations have conducted and published the results of a number of studies relevant to nursing practice in the context of the health care system. The two prevalent themes of these studies have been quality and safety.

In its 2000 report *To Err Is Human: Building a Safer Health System*, the IOM discussed the issue of errors in hospitals, estimating that as many as 98,000 hospitalized Americans die each year not as a result of their illness or disease, but as a result of errors in their care. That report was followed closely in 2001 by an IOM report entitled *Crossing the Quality Chasm: A New Health System for the 21st Century* that identified health care quality issues, called for a radical redesign of the U.S. health care system, and proposed six quality outcomes: safety, effectiveness, patient-centeredness, timeliness, efficiency, and equity. This report also emphasized that safety and quality issues are more often the result of systems issues than of individual performance. The *Crossing the Quality Chasm* report was followed in 2003 by *Health Professions Education: A Bridge to Quality,* which focused on integrating a core set of competencies into the education of all health professionals. The five core competencies for all clinicians are:

1. Provide patient-centered care.

2. Work in interdisciplinary teams.

3. Employ evidence-based practice.

4. Apply quality improvement.

5. Utilize informatics (IOM, 2003).

The Agency for Healthcare Research and Quality (AHRQ) then asked the IOM to conduct a study to identify key aspects of the work environment for nurses that likely have an impact on patient safety and potential improvements in health care working conditions that would likely increase patient safety. As a result, the IOM in 2004 specifically addressed the role of nursing and the nursing work environment in assuring patient safety in *Keeping Patients Safe: Transforming the Work Environment of Nurses.*

In early 2007, the Robert Wood Johnson Foundation (RWJF) funded an initiative called Quality and Safety Education for Nurses (QSEN) to address "the challenge of preparing nurses with the competencies necessary to continuously improve the quality and safety of the health care systems in which they work" (Cronenwett et al., 2007, p. 122). The QSEN team adapted the competencies from the IOM (2003) *Health Professions Education* report for nursing (see Table 1.3) and delineated the knowledge, skills, and attitudes for each competency. The QSEN competencies, which were first designed to be used in schools of nursing, are now permeating all sites where nurses practice.

Quality and safety are two major parts of the context in which nurses practice and, as such, are critical to precepting. In looking at the QSEN competencies, you can easily see how they could also be applied to precepting itself—for example, recognizing the preceptee as a partner and assuring the safety of the preceptee and of the patient.

Table 1.3   Quality and Safety Education for Nurses
Patient-Centered Care
Recognize the patient or designee as the source of control and full partner in providing compassionate care based on respect for patient's preferences, values, and needs.
Teamwork and Collaboration
Function effectively within nursing and interprofessional teams, fostering open communication, mutual respect, and shared decision-making to achieve quality patient care.
Evidence-based Practice
Integrate best current evidence with clinical expertise and patient/family preferences and values for delivery of optimal health care.
Quality Improvement
Use data to monitor the outcomes of care processes and use improvement methods to design and test changes to continuously improve the quality and safety of health care systems.
Safety
Minimize the risk of harm to patients though both system effectiveness and individual performance.
Informatics
Use information and technology to communicate, manage knowledge, mitigate error, and support decision-making.

Source: Cronenwett et al., 2007

Most recently, with the goal of improving how health care is delivered to better meet the needs of all patients, the IOM and the RWJF partnered on a landmark initiative on the future of nursing to assure that nurses are well-positioned to lead change and advance health (IOM, 2010). Four key messages structure the discussion and recommendations presented in their report:

1. Nurses should practice to the full extent of their education and training.

2. Nurses should achieve higher levels of education and training through an improved education system that promotes seamless academic progression.

3. Nurses should be full partners, with physicians and other health professionals, in redesigning health care in the United States.

4. Effective workforce planning and policymaking require better data collection and an improved information structure.

The specific recommendations from the IOM/RWJF initiative on the future of nursing are shown in Table 1.4. Many of the recommendations have direct implications for preceptors. Ongoing information on state and national activities designed to implement the recommendations can be found at *http://thefutureofnursing.org.*

Table 1.4   Recommendations From *The Future of Nursing* Initiative

- **Remove scope-of-practice barriers.** Advanced practice registered nurses should be able to practice to the full extent of their education and training.

- **Expand opportunities for nurses to lead and diffuse collaborative improvement efforts.** Private and public funders, health care organizations, nursing education programs, and nursing associations should expand opportunities for nurses to lead and manage collaborative efforts with physicians and other members of the health care team to conduct research and to redesign and improve practice environments and health systems. These entities should also provide opportunities for nurses to diffuse successful practices.

- **Implement nurse residency programs.** State boards of nursing, accrediting bodies, the federal government, and health care organizations should take actions to support nurses' completion of a transition-to-practice program (nurse residency) after they have completed a prelicensure or advanced practice degree program or when they are transitioning into new clinical practice areas.

- **Increase the proportion of nurses with a baccalaureate degree to 80% by 2020.** Academic nurse leaders across all schools of nursing should work together to increase the proportion of nurses with a baccalaureate degree from 50% to 80% by 2020. These leaders should partner with education accrediting bodies, private and public funders, and employers to ensure funding, monitor progress, and increase the diversity of students to create a workforce prepared to meet the demands of diverse populations across the lifespan.

- **Double the number of nurses with a doctorate by 2020.** Schools of nursing, with support from private and public funders, academic administrators and university trustees, and accrediting bodies, should double the number of nurses with a doctorate by 2020 to add to the cadre of nurse faculty and researchers, with attention to increasing diversity.

- **Ensure that nurses engage in lifelong learning.** Accrediting bodies, schools of nursing, health care organizations, and continuing competency educators from multiple health professions should collaborate to ensure that nurses and nursing students and faculty continue their education and engage in lifelong learning to gain the competencies needed to provide care for diverse populations across the lifespan.

Table 1.4   Recommendations From *The Future of Nursing* Initiative (cont.)
• **Prepare and enable nurses to lead change to advance health.** Nurses, nursing education programs, and nursing associations should prepare the nursing workforce to assume leadership positions across all levels, while public, private, and governmental health care decision makers should ensure that leadership positions are available to and filled by nurses.
• **Build an infrastructure for the collection and analysis of interprofessional health care workforce data.** The National Health Care Workforce Commission, with oversight from the Government Accountability Office and the Health Resources and Services Administration, should lead a collaborative effort to improve research and the collection and analysis of data on health care workforce requirements. The Workforce Commission and the Health Resources and Services Administration should collaborate with state licensing boards, state nursing workforce centers, and the Department of Labor in this effort to ensure that the data are timely and publicly accessible.

Source: IOM, 2010

Preceptor Roles

Preceptors have many roles: teacher/coach, leader/influencer, facilitator, evaluator, socialization agent, protector, and role model.

Teacher/Coach

The teacher/coach role is the one most people think of when they think of precepting. Regardless of whether a preceptee is a new graduate nurse or an experienced nurse going into a new field, the preceptee comes to the preceptor to learn something the preceptor knows, and to enhance or expand the preceptee's knowledge and expertise. Preceptors need to understand not only the science of teaching (learning theories, etc.) but also the art of teaching (how to apply the science in a way that is effective). Ohrling and Hallberg (2000) found four themes critical to preceptees' learning:

1. Creating a space for learning

2. Providing concrete illustrations

3. Providing control over the opportunities and pace of learning

4. Allowing time for reflection

The coaching role takes teaching one step further. It's not just about learning the skill; it's about how and when to use the skill and how to use it most effectively. That's where the coaching comes in. It also comes in when preceptees have a difficult time grasping what is being taught or, on the other end of the spectrum, show the potential to move to a higher level of performance.

Leader/Influencer

Preceptors are leaders and influencers. Leadership is expected of all registered nurses (ANA, 2010b), but especially those who precept others. Often, people incorrectly believe that leadership and influence only come with authority. Generally, preceptors do not have line authority over the preceptees or others who are needed to assist in the preceptors' work with the preceptees. Cohen and Bradford (2005) developed an influence without authority model using reciprocity and exchange that can be helpful to preceptors. The key aspects of the model are:

- Assume that everyone is a potential ally.
- Clarify your goals and priorities—know what you want.
- Diagnose the world of other people—their goals, concerns, and needs.
- Identify relevant currencies—what do you each value?
- Deal with relationships—both the nature of your current relationship and how the person wants to be related to.
- Influence through give and take.

Preceptors can use their influence in many situations to obtain what is needed in their roles as preceptors and nurses.

Another way that preceptors lead and influence is through their values. The American Association of Colleges of Nursing (2008) has identified five values that epitomize the caring, professional nurse:

1. Altruism (a concern for the welfare and well-being of others)

2. Autonomy (right to self-determination)

3. Human dignity (respect for the inherent worth and uniqueness of individuals and populations)

4. Integrity (acting in accordance with a code of ethics and standards of practice)

5. Social justice (fair treatment)

Some values are more specific; for example, timeliness, job security, peer support, and recognition. It is important to understand what you value and what others value. You can influence the values of another individual without any intention to do so. Therefore, preceptors must understand the values they convey by their words and their actions.

Preceptors also need to identify when values conflicts occur. This can sometimes be especially difficult for new graduate nurses to deal with; for example, in situations in which what the patient or family wants or values conflicts with what the new graduate nurse values or wants. A significant inverse correlation has been found between value congruence and quality care, and between value congruence and nurse job satisfaction (Kramer & Hafner, 1989), making the need to resolve values differences important for both patient care outcomes and nurse retention.

Values

What do you value?

What does your manager value?

What does your organization value?

What does your preceptee value?

Facilitator

Preceptors are constantly facilitating, whether it's finding assignments that meet the needs of preceptees or making connections between preceptees and other departments. At the beginning of the preceptor-preceptee relationship, preceptors facilitate more. As preceptees progress, they can assume more of the facilitation responsibility.

A key goal of the facilitating role is creating a positive and rich learning environment for the preceptee. John Dewey (1925), an American educational reformer who emphasized pragmatism, the teacher's role as a facilitator and guide, and the need for experiential learning, said, "No one with an honest respect for scientific conclusions can deny that experience is something that occurs only under highly specialized conditions, such as are found in a highly organized creature which in turn requires a specialized environment. There is no evidence that experience occurs everywhere and everywhen" (p. 3a). Experiential learning requires an environment in which the experiences, and the learning that occurs from those experiences, are intentionally planned.

Evaluator

Evaluation is often a new skill for preceptors. It is not an easy thing to evaluate the performance of another, especially when the person's job rests on your evaluation. Evaluation is made easier for the evaluator and the evaluatee by the presence of criteria-based competencies. In other words, you both know the outcomes and standards that need to be met before you begin the process. As will be discussed in Chapter 4, preceptors need to separate teaching and coaching activities from evaluation activities so that the learner is free to learn during the time designated for teaching and coaching.

A major aspect of evaluating is providing feedback and constructive criticism to reinforce good performance, correct poor performance, and understand how improvements can be made. Cantillon and Sargeant (2008) provide nine general principles for effective feedback:

1. Feedback should be viewed as a normal, everyday component of the teacher-learner relationship, so that both sides can expect it and manage its effects.

2. Learners should be clear about the criteria against which their performance will be assessed.

3. Feedback should be given on specific behaviors rather than on general performance.

4. Feedback should be based on what is directly observed.

5. Feedback should be phrased in nonjudgmental language.

6. Timeliness of feedback is important. Feedback should be given at the time of the event or shortly afterward.

7. Feedback should be limited to one or two items.

8. Feedback from the teacher should be balanced by deliberately seeking the learners' perceptions of their performance and their ideas about how to improve it.

9. Feedback should lead to changes in the learner's thinking, behavior, and performance.

In addition, whenever possible, feedback should be given in private and in a setting that is free from distraction.

Socialization Agent

Hinshaw (1977) defines socialization as "the process of learning new roles and the adaptation to them, and, as such, continual processes by which individuals become members of a social group" (p. 2). Preceptors facilitate the socialization of preceptees into the organization, into the unit, and even into the nursing shift within a unit by teaching preceptees the norms, the "sacred cows," the formal and informal expectations, and the unwritten rules of the game. For new graduate nurses, preceptors also facilitate socialization into the profession. In addition, preceptors can influence others to be accepting of and encouraging to preceptees.

Socialization is particularly important with new graduate nurses. As Kramer (1974) noted in *Reality Shock*, the seminal work on new graduate transition, "it seems that the socialization that takes place in medical and nursing schools prepares students to be medical and nursing students, but not physicians and nurses" (p. 42). It is the job of the preceptors to socialize new graduate nurses into the professional nursing role.

Protector

Preceptors are protectors of both patients and preceptees. The number one concern in precepting is assuring a safe environment for patients. Preceptors have to find or create situations in which preceptees can learn while at the same time protecting the safety of patients. There should never be any doubt that patient safety is job one.

Creating a safe learning environment for preceptees is also the responsibility of preceptors. Creating a safe learning environment begins with making sure that preceptees feel safe in asking questions. The message that "there are no dumb questions" is important. Preceptees must be able to freely express their lack of understanding, their doubts about their competence, etc., so that these issues can be addressed in a professional and timely manner.

Creating a safe learning environment also includes protecting preceptees from disruptive behavior and lateral/horizontal (nurse on nurse) violence. Two recent studies revealed that 17% of the verbal abuse experienced by critical care nurses came from other RNs (Ulrich et al., 2006, 2009). Preceptors must protect preceptees and, at the same time, teach them how to deal with these types of behaviors.

Modic and Schoessler (2008) suggest the following strategies for minimizing horizontal violence:

- Be alert to behaviors that indicate horizontal violence or bullying is going on.

- Be aware that the preceptee, especially if a new graduate, is in a vulnerable position.

- Be aware of your own behavior. Model professional behaviors.

- If you see bullying or incivility, point out the behavior to the individual in a respectful manner.

- Help preceptees learn how to speak up.

- Talk to the manager or others in authority about your concerns.

- Talk with your colleagues about how to create a healthier work environment.

Role Model

Preceptors role model competencies and professional practice. Preceptors must have demonstrated competence in the roles they are precepting. Preceptees will quickly notice if there is dissonance between what the preceptor tells them to do and what they see the preceptor doing. Though there might be more than one way to accomplish a task that results in the same outcome, preceptees do not have the experience to know that and will be confused if you tell them one thing and do another, or if they see other nurses doing a task in a way that is different from how they have been taught. Preceptors also need to make other staff aware that they too are role models for the preceptees. As with evaluations, role modeling is easier if everyone adheres to the same standards of practice and professional performance. As this is not always what occurs, preceptors need to be prepared to explain the conflicts to preceptees.

Conclusion

Precepting occurs in the context of quality and safety in nursing and health care. Through a myriad of roles, preceptors work with preceptees to move them from novices to experts and to assure that they are competent to care for patients and perform their roles. Being a preceptor involves understanding the context in which nurses practice and learning the aspects of all of the preceptor roles.

References

American Association of Colleges of Nursing. (2008). *The essentials of baccalaureate education for professional nursing practice.* Washington, DC: Author.

American Nurses Association. (ANA). (2001). *Code of ethics for nurses with interpretive statements.* Silver Spring, MD: Author.

American Nurses Association. (ANA). (2010a). *Nursing's social policy statement: The essence of the profession.* Silver Spring, MD: Author.

American Nurses Association (ANA). (2010b). *Nursing: Scope and standards of practice* (2nd ed.). Silver Spring, MD: Author.

Cantillon, P., & Sargeant, J. (2008). Giving feedback in clinical settings. *British Medical Journal, 337,* 1292-1294.

Cohen, A. R., & Bradford, D. L. (2005). *Influence without authority.* Hoboken, NJ: John Wiley & Sons.

Cronenwett, L., Sherwood, G., Barnsteiner, J., Disch, J., Johnson, J., Mitchell, P., Warren, J. (2007). Quality and safety education for nurses. *Nursing Outlook, 35*(3), 122-131.

Dewey, J. (1925). *Experience and nature.* London: Open Court Publishing Company.

Hinshaw, A. S. (1977). Socialization and resocialization of nurses for professional nursing practice. In L. Netzer (Ed.), *Education, administration, and change* (pp. 1-15). New York, NY: National League for Nursing.

Institute of Medicine (IOM). (2000). *To err is human: Building a safer health system.* Washington, DC: National Academies Press.

Institute of Medicine (IOM). (2001). *Crossing the quality chasm: A new health system for the 21st century.* Washington, DC: National Academies Press.

Institute of Medicine (IOM). (2003). *Health professions education: A bridge to quality.* Washington, DC: National Academies Press.

Institute of Medicine (IOM). (2004). *Keeping patients safe: Transforming the work environment of nurses.* Washington, DC: National Academies Press.

Institute of Medicine (IOM). Committee on the Robert Wood Johnson Foundation initiative on the future of nursing. (2010). *The future of nursing: Leading change, advocating health.* Washington, DC: National Academies Press.

Kramer, M. (1974). *Reality shock: Why nurses leave nursing.* St. Louis, MO: C.V. Mosby Company.

Kramer, M., & Hafner, L. P. (1989). Shared values: Impact on staff nurse job satisfaction and perceived productivity. *Nursing Research, 38*(3), 172-177.

Modic, M. B., & Schoessler, M. (2008). Preceptorship: The role of the preceptor in minimizing horizontal violence. *Journal for Nurses in Staff Development, 24*(4), 189-190.

Ohrling, K., & Hallberg, I. R. (2000). Student nurses' lived experience of preceptorship. Part 2: The preceptor-preceptee relationship. *International Journal of Nursing Students, 37*(1), 25-36.

Ulrich, B. T., Lavandero, R., Hart, K., Woods, D., Leggett, J., & Taylor, D. (2006). Critical care nurses' work environments: A baseline status report. *Critical Care Nurse, 26*(5), 46-57.

Ulrich, B. T., Lavandero, R., Hart, K. A., Woods, D., Leggett, J., Friedman, D., D'Aurizio, P., & Edwards, S. J. (2009). Critical care nurses' work environments 2008: A follow-up report. *Critical Care Nurse, 29*(2), 93-

Preceptor Development Plan: Preceptor Roles

Think about each of the roles of a preceptor. What are your strengths in each role? In which areas do you need to increase your knowledge and expertise? What is your plan for expanding your knowledge and expertise? What resources are available? Who can help you?

Name:			
Role: Teacher/Coach			
Strengths	Needs	Plan	Resources
Role: Leader/Influencer			
Strengths	Needs	Plan	Resources
Role: Facilitator			
Strengths	Needs	Plan	Resources
Role: Evaluator			
Strengths	Needs	Plan	Resources
Role: Socialization Agent			
Strengths	Needs	Plan	Resources
Role: Protector			
Strengths	Needs	Plan	Resources
Role: Role Model			
Strengths	Needs	Plan	Resources

Note: This form and other resources are available at www.RNPreceptor.com.

"Knowledge is power, and professional practice means a lifetime commitment to learning."

–Luther Christman

Learning: The Foundation of Precepting

2

Beth Tamplet Ulrich, EdD, RN, FACHE, FAAN

OBJECTIVES

- Understand assumptions about adult learners

- Understand the concepts of observing and modeling and how they apply to preceptor behavior and preceptee learning

- Apply the novice to expert framework to both preceptor and preceptee learning

- Understand learning styles

Learning is a component of precepting that might sound simple, but it requires a great deal of attention from preceptors. To successfully work with preceptees, preceptors need an understanding of learning theories, models, and styles. The information in this chapter provides an overview of adult learning theory, transformative learning theory, social learning theory, Maslow's hierarchy of needs, Benner's novice to expert model, and learning styles. Understanding how learning occurs and is facilitated is the foundation of precepting.

Adult Learning Theory

Malcolm Knowles is generally recognized as the father of adult learning. Knowles believed that adults learn differently than children and that adult learners possess unique characteristics. To differentiate adult learning from pedagogy (the art and science of teaching children), he used the term *andragogy* (from the Greek words *aner* meaning "man" and *agogus* meaning "the leader of"; Knowles, 1973). Knowles' work also shifted the focus of learning from the teacher to the learner. In adult learning, the learner's experience counts as much as the teacher's knowledge. In some adult learning situations, it even becomes difficult to determine whether the teacher or the student is learning more (Knowles, Holton, & Swanson, 2005).

Knowles (1973) began with four assumptions about the adult learner and later added two more (Knowles, 1984, 1987; see Table 2.1). The assumptions are:

1. Need to know—Adults need to know why they need to learn something.

2. Self-concept—As individuals mature, they have increasing self-directedness.

3. The role of experience—As individuals mature, they accumulate experiences that cause them to be an increasingly rich resource for learning and also provide them with a broadening base on which to relate new learning.

4. Readiness to learn—As individuals mature, their readiness to learn becomes a product of their perceived need to learn.

5. Orientation to learning—Adults have a problem-centered approach to learning. They want to learn a particular competency or acquire knowledge that they can apply immediately to an identified problem.

6. Motivation—Adult learners are internally motivated.

Table 2.1   Core Adult Learning Principles
• Learner's need to know: why, what, how
• Self-concept of learner: autonomous, self-directed
• Prior experience of learner: resource, mental models
• Readiness to learn: life-related, developmental task
• Orientation to learning: problem-centered, contextual
• Motivation to learn: intrinsic value, personal payoff

Source: Knowles, Holton, & Swanson, 1998

It should be noted, however, that Knowles did not believe that all of his assumptions about adult learning must be utilized in all situations. Rather, he believed that an essential feature of the model was its flexibility, and he encouraged adaptation based on the purpose of the learning event.

Holton, Swanson, and Naquin (2001) reviewed Knowles' adult learning theory and subsequent research on adult learning. They concluded that the biggest advancement in the understanding of adult learning since the work of Knowles was the research on how individual differences of learners affect adult learning, and they expressed their belief that understanding individual differences makes Knowles' adult learning theory more effective. Individual differences have been described in three main areas:

1. Cognitive—General mental abilities, primary mental abilities, cognitive controls, cognitive styles in information gathering and information organizing, and learning styles

2. Personality—Attentional and engagement styles and expectancy and incentive styles

3. Prior knowledge (Jonassen & Grabowski, 1993)

Knowledge of the individual differences can be used to individualize adult learning experiences in a variety of ways.

Knowles, Holton, and Swanson (1998) created what they termed the andragogy in practice model, which incorporated Knowles' adult learning assumptions with individual and situational differences and the goals and purposes for learning. Holton and colleagues (2001) then suggested the following approach for adult learners using the andragogy in practice model:

- Use Knowles' assumptions to form the foundation for planning adult learning experiences.

- Conduct analyses to understand "a) the particular adult learners and their individual characteristics, b) the characteristics of the subject matter, and c) the characteristics of the particular situation in which adult learning is being used" (p. 136) and anticipate adjustments to the assumptions.

- Use the goals and purposes for which the learning is conducted to provide a frame that shapes the learning experience.

Preceptors can use the andragogy in practice model to apply adult learning theory, assess the learner's readiness to learn and prior experience, and create meaningful learning experiences that encourage learner engagement. Nursing students at both undergraduate and graduate levels and practicing nurses have had experience with at least some hands-on learning. However, given the limited clinical time in nursing education, the experience might not have been long enough or in enough depth to allow nursing students to apply their theoretical knowledge.

Knowledge of adult learning theory can help preceptors understand their preceptees and create more meaningful learning experiences for them. Preceptors can create situations in which preceptees can use what they learn immediately—a scenario that is attractive to adult learners. Such immediate use is advantageous, because if adult learners begin to acquire a new skill but then do not have the opportunity to practice it, the skill competency fades quickly (Zemke & Zemke, 1995).

Transformative Learning Theory

Transformative learning theory complements and supports adult learning theory. Transformative learning, according to Mezirow (1997, p. 5) is "the process of effecting change in a frame of reference." It is based on the premise that all individuals have perspectives derived from their experiences, thoughts, values, and insights (Mezirow, 1991).

Transformative learning has three aspects: experience, critical reflection, and development (Merriam & Caffarella, 1999). A learner's experience, which is also one of Knowles' adult learning assumptions, forms the basis for future learning. Critical reflection, part of Knowles' self-directedness assumption, is an integral part of transformative learning, because the learner needs time and often encouragement to contemplate and reflect on how the new learning fits with past experience (Lieb, 1991). Development is a necessary ongoing process in transformational learning.

To facilitate transformational learning, preceptors must help preceptees become aware and critical of the assumptions and experiences of themselves and others. Preceptees must be encouraged to view problems and new information from different perspectives. For this to occur, preceptors need to create positive learning environments in which preceptees feel safe in trying out new thoughts and critical reflections. Preceptors should encourage and support discourse.

Social Learning Theory

Social learning theory emphasizes learning through observing and modeling (Bandura, 1969, 1977). Of special interest to nursing is Bandura's (1969) finding that modeling is "an indispensable means of transmitting and modifying behavior in situations where errors are likely to produce costly or fatal consequences" (p. 213).

Several conditions must be met for the observing and modeling to occur:

- Attention—In order to learn, an individual must be attentive to the behavior being modeled.

- Retention—Retention involves the ability to retain information about the behavior that was observed.

- Reproduction—Reproduction of the behavior relies on having observed all components of the behavior as well as having the ability to perform the behavior.

- Motivation—The learner has to have a good reason to do the observed behavior. Individuals are more likely to adopt a behavior if they value the outcome of performing the behavior.

Preceptors should note that the observation and modeling of behaviors are not limited to those behaviors that preceptees should model. Being a preceptor is akin to having a video recording of everything you do implanted in the preceptee's brain. It becomes the responsibility of preceptors to critically reflect on their own behaviors and to assure that what the preceptees observe is what should be modeled.

Hierarchy of Needs Theory

Maslow's hierarchy of needs theory has applicability in both precepting and patient care. Maslow's original hierarchy of needs (the one most people are familiar with) contained five levels of basic needs that Maslow believed every individual attempts to attain:

- Biological and physiological needs—hunger, thirst

- Safety needs—safety, security

- Belongingness and love needs—affiliating with others, being accepted

- Esteem needs—achievement, competence, recognition

- Self-actualization—fulfillment, reaching one's potential (Maslow, 1954)

These needs were based on the premise that an individual would be ready to act on higher-level growth needs only if the basic needs were met.

In Maslow's subsequent work, he expanded the hierarchy of needs to include eight levels (see Figure 2.1; Maslow, 1971; Maslow & Lowery, 1998). He added two levels below self-actualization—the cognitive need to know, understand, and explore; and the aesthetic need for order, symmetry, and beauty. Above self-actualization, he added self-transcendence—the need to connect with something beyond one's ego and to help others find self-fulfillment and realize their potential. Maslow also noted that while striving for higher levels of need, individuals can enjoy experiences along the way: "Achieving basic-need gratifications gives us many peak experiences, each of which are absolute delights, perfect in themselves, and needing no more than themselves to validate life" (Maslow & Lowery, 1998, pp. 169-170).

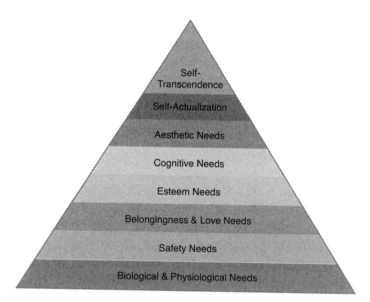

Figure 2.1   Maslow's hierarchy of needs

Adapted from Maslow & Lowery, 1998.

At the most basic level of Maslow's hierarchy of needs, preceptors need to assure that preceptees feel safe in their practice environment. After that is attended to, preceptors can then help preceptees move up the hierarchy. Preceptors themselves can find self-actualization and even self-transcendence in the act of precepting others.

From Novice to Expert

Patricia Benner's (1984) landmark work on the novice to expert model of how nurses acquire skills and knowledge forms the foundation of many nursing school curricula and of many hospital-based preceptorship programs. Benner applied the Dreyfus model of skill acquisition to nursing. The Dreyfus model, developed by Stuart and Hubert Dreyfus (1980) after studying airline pilots, chess players, and individuals who were learning languages, is comprised of a five-level proficiency hierarchy of skill acquisition and development. Benner (1984) notes that the levels reflect changes in three aspects:

- Movement from reliance on abstract principles to use of past concrete experience as paradigms

- Change in the learner's perception of the demand situation from equally relevant bits to a whole with only some relevant parts

- Passage from detached observer to involved performer

The levels are novice, advanced beginner, competent, proficient, and expert (see Table 2.2). Experiential learning is essential to progress from the novice to expert level. The preceptor can tailor the learning experiences by recognizing the level of the preceptee and understanding the progression needed through the levels to attain the skills and knowledge needed to move toward expert practice. This process is discussed in detail in future chapters.

Table 2.2   Novice to Expert

	Novice	Advanced Beginner	Competent	Proficient	Expert
Experience	None	Minimal	Moderate, specific	Moderate, broad	Extensive
Recollection	Non-situational	Situational	Situational	Situational	Situational
Recognition	Decomposed	Decomposed	Holistic	Holistic	Holistic
Decision	Analytical	Analytical	Analytical	Intuitive	Intuitive
Awareness	Monitoring	Monitoring	Monitoring	Monitoring	Absorbed
Information	Little understanding of contextual meaning	Beginning to see contextual meaning	Sees patterns and begins to discriminate relevance	Prioritizes information	Deep understanding of total situation

Table 2.2	Novice to Expert (cont.)				
	Novice	*Advanced Beginner*	*Competent*	*Proficient*	*Expert*
Behavior	Rule-governed, inflexible	Uses more sophisticated rules. Begins to identify conditional rules	Begins to devise new rules and reasoning procedures	Involved, intuitive response	Sees what needs to be done and does it; trusts intuition
Responsibility for Outcomes	Low responsibility	Low responsibility	Responsible for own decisions and practice	Sense of responsibility increases	Responsible and seeks to improve. Extends responsibility to others and organization

Adapted from Benner, 1984; Benner, Tanner, & Chelsa, 2009; Dreyfus & Dreyfus, 1980, 2009

Learning Is Facilitated . . .

- In an atmosphere that encourages the learner to be an active participant in the process

- In an atmosphere that provides opportunities for the learner to discover the personal meaning of ideas

- When the learner feels that his or her ideas, feelings, and perspectives have value and significance

- In an atmosphere in which different ideas can be accepted (but not necessarily agreed with). Situations that emphasize the "the one right answer" or a "magical solution" limit exploration and inhibit discovery.

- In an atmosphere where the learner's right to make mistakes is recognized

- In an atmosphere that encourages openness of self rather than concealment of self

- When learners are encouraged to trust themselves, as originators of ideas, and to share their ideas with others

- In an atmosphere that permits free and open communication and confrontation

Source: Lore, 1981

The novice to expert model is situational. A nurse can be at the expert level in one area of nursing and at the novice level in another. For example, a nurse who is learning to become a preceptor might be a novice or advanced beginner in precepting yet be an expert in a clinical specialty. Likewise, an experienced nurse entering a new clinical specialty has certain skills, knowledge, and experience on which to build expertise in the new specialty, but both the experienced nurse and the preceptor must assess what is known and applicable and what is yet to be learned.

Learning Styles

Individuals are different in many ways, including how they learn. Not everyone learns or learns best in the same way, or learns best in the same way in all situations. In the quest to continually improve learning, and concomitantly teaching, many approaches to determining learning styles have been developed. It is not necessary to choose or prefer one style over the others. Multiple style concepts can occur simultaneously or sequentially.

Preceptors can use the awareness gained from an overview of learning style concepts to better understand the needs and preferences of individual preceptees and to better provide information and experiences to the preceptees in ways that have the best chance of being effective and efficient. Opinions are mixed on whether it is beneficial to encourage preceptees to move out of the comfort of their preferred styles to learn new styles, thereby expanding their future options. Like many other things, the best approach might be a progression— starting with using the preferred style for novices and adding new styles to their repertoire as novices acquire skills and knowledge.

The ways individuals learn are sometimes referred to as learning theories (although some are not theories), learning styles (although some are not styles), learning preferences, learning models and constructs, or by many other names. Regardless of the name, the main interest in how people learn emanates from wanting to know how individuals receive and process information, how they store information in the brain, and how they retrieve and use it. Though many learning style concepts exist, each of the concepts has in common an acknowledgement of the diversity among learners.

Characteristics of Styles

Styles ...

Are preferences, not abilities

Are not good or bad

Can vary across tasks and situations

Are socialized

Can vary across the life span

Are measurable

Are modifiable

Source: Sternberg, 1997

Curry's Learning Style Classification System

Curry (1983, 1987) developed a classification system for learning styles, describing the system as being like layers of an onion. The innermost core layer is cognitive personality styles, a relatively permanent personality dimension that addresses an individual's approach to adopting and assimilating information. The next layer is information processing styles, followed by the layer of social interaction. The outermost layer is instructional preferences—how the learner interacts with the learning environment and with instructional practices, and the learner's preference of the environment in which to learn. Instructional preferences are seen as the least stable and the most easily influenced layer.

Cognitive Styles

Cognitive styles describe an individual's approach to acquiring, adapting, assimilating, and processing information. Merriam and Caffarella (1999) have described cognitive styles as "consistencies in information processing that develop with underlying personality traits" (p. 11). Cognitive styles are seen as an underlying and relatively permanent personality dimension that affects more than learning.

Gregorc's Learning Styles

Gregorc (1979) studied how learners perceive and order new information. He believed that "the human mind has channels through which it receives and expresses information most efficiently and effectively" (Gregorc, 1982, p. 5). He found that information is acquired through either abstract or concrete processes, or a combination of both, and that arranging, prioritizing, and using that information occur by random or sequential ordering patterns. Gregorc believed that these tendencies—abstract, concrete, random, and sequential—reflect inborn predispositions, but he also felt that individuals need to be able to function in ways other than their natural style.

Gregorc (1979, 1984) identified four learning styles: concrete sequential, concrete random, abstract sequential, and abstract random.

1. Concrete sequential learners prefer learning that is direct, orderly (step-by-step instructions), and hands-on—for example, workbooks and computer instruction.

2. Concrete random learners prefer trial and error, flexibility, and problem solving—for example, simulation and independent study.

3. Abstract sequential learners prefer analytic, logical approaches—for example, group discussion.

4. Abstract random learners prefer holistic, unstructured learning—for example, lectures and reading.

Myers-Briggs

The Myers-Briggs Type Indicator (MBTI), developed in 1962, is one of the oldest and longstanding assessment instruments to describe personality traits. It is based on the theory of personality types developed by Carl Jung (Myers & McCaulley, 1985). The MBTI identifies four dichotomous dimensions/preferences:

1. Extroversion (outward turning)—Introversion (inward turning)

2. Sensing (looks for facts)—Intuitive (looks for meaning)

3. Thinking (uses objective data)—Feeling (uses subjective data)

4. Judgment (ordered)—Perception (flexible and open)

Sixteen different combinations of the dimensions/preferences are possible, but because most preceptees will not have taken the MBTI, preceptors can best use the four dimensions/preferences of the MBTI to raise their awareness of ways in which the preceptees might learn better.

Field Dependence/Independence

Witkin and colleagues (1971) studied individual differences in perception and spatial awareness. Their major finding related to field dependence/independence, the degree to which an individual "uses context in order to understand and make sense of new information" (Smith, 2002, p. 65). In other words, does the individual need the context to better identify new information? Can the individual see new information as separate from the field surrounding it, or must the information be immersed in the surrounding field to be seen? Some nurses are known among their peers as being able to spot key observations about patients regardless of the setting and the distractions that are around the patient; such nurses would be described as field independent. In sports, a quarterback who always seems to spot the open receiver would also be said to be field independent. The quarterback sees the receiver regardless of what's around him or the receiver.

It also seems that learners process information differently based on their field independence/dependence. Learners who are field independent tend to be more analytical and logical; are less influenced by authority, social attachments, and external standards; and tend to be intrinsically motivated and guided by their own values. Field dependent learners tend to have a less defined sense of autonomy and independence and are extrinsically motivated, relying on an external frame of reference for information and guidance (Jonassen & Grabowski, 1993). Field independence and field dependence can be measured using an embedded figures test, but can also be observed by astute preceptors. Given the chaos and number of people who can sometimes surround a patient and the interruptions that frequently occur in a hospital while trying to deliver patient care, it is important for preceptors to help preceptees develop field independence.

Information Processing Styles

Information processing styles reflect an individual's preferred approach to assimilating information. Kolb (1984) based his work on what he called experiential learning, believing that experience is the source of learning and development. He described experiential learning as "the process whereby knowledge is created through the transformation of experience. Knowledge results from the combination of grasping experience and transforming it" (p. 41). He described the characteristics of experiential learning:

- A continuous holistic process of adaptation to the world

- Grounded in experience

- Involves transactions between the learner and the environment

- Full of tension

- A process of creating knowledge that results from the transaction between social knowledge and personal knowledge

Kolb identified two continuums of learning: the processing continuum (doing/watching: the learner's approach to a task) and the perception continuum (feeling/thinking: the learner's emotional response). Using these two continuums, Kolb developed a learning cycle with four points:

1. Concrete experience (feeling; learning from specific experiences and relating to people)

2. Reflective observation (watching; looking for the meaning in things)

3. Abstract conceptualization (thinking; logically analyzing ideas and acting on an intellectual understanding)

4. Active experimentation (doing; getting things done by influencing people and events; risk-taking)

Each quadrant of the learning cycle represented a learning style:

- Diverging—feeling and watching

- Assimilating—thinking and watching

- Converging—thinking and doing

- Accommodating—feeling and doing

Learners can enter the cyclical learning process at any point. Kolb believes that they learn a task best if they practice all four modes, moving and balancing between concrete experience and abstract conceptualization and between reflective observation and active experimentation. Kolb believes that learning styles are not fixed personality traits, but rather are stable patterns of behavior based on the learner's background and experience. Kolb's Learning Style Inventory (Kolb, 1999) is the most widely used information processing assessment tool.

Instructional Preferences

Dunn and Dunn (1978) studied how individuals prefer to learn and developed a learning style concept that includes environmental, sociological, emotional, psychological, and physical preferences:

- Environmental (sound, temperature, lighting, formality of setting, etc.).

- Sociological (whether the learner prefers to learn alone or in groups, with authority figures present or not, or through routine or variety).

- Emotional (the learner's motivation, persistence, and need for structure).

- Psychological (how learners process information—analytical/global, right brain/ left brain, impulsive/reflective)

- Physical (perceptual strengths—verbal, visual, tactile, kinesthetic, time of day, need for mobility.

By understanding how preceptees prefer to learn, preceptors can tailor to their preferences when possible.

Sensory Learning Styles

Sensory learning styles include visual, auditory, tactile, and kinesthetic. Visual learners prefer reading written materials and seeing pictures. Auditory learners would do well listening to podcasts. Tactile learners need to touch—to have hands on. Kinesthetic learners immerse themselves. People often give you cues in conversation to their preferred sensory style: "I see what you mean." "I hear what you say." "I feel your pain."

Sensory styles apply to more than learning. It's good to know, for example, how your boss likes to receive information. Does he or she want to meet and talk about it? Does your boss prefer to read the details? Or, is a picture really worth a thousand words?

Conclusion: Preceptor as Learner and Preceptor as Teacher

Preceptors can use the information in this chapter in two ways. As a learner, you should critically reflect on your own learning and your own experience. What do you need to learn to be a competent, proficient, and then an expert preceptor? What experience do you have that will be applicable? What is your frame of reference? Are you ready to learn?

As a teacher, this chapter's information can form the foundation of how you approach preceptees and the learning experiences that you develop for them. Who will you be precepting? Undergraduate nursing students? New graduate nurses? Experienced nurses entering a new specialty? Each will have different needs. How will you model for them what they need to learn?

To be a successful preceptor, you must begin by understanding learning. Also, when you learn a new role, such as precepting, you will find it helpful to understand how you yourself learn best. The theories and models presented in this chapter form the foundation on which preceptor competence is built.

References

Bandura, A. (1969). Social-learning theory of identificory processes. In D. A. Goslin (Ed.), *Handbook of socialization theory and research* (pp. 213-262). New York: Rand McNally & Co.

Bandura, A. (1977). *Social learning theory.* New York: General Learning Press.

Benner, P. (1984). *From novice to expert: Excellence and power in clinical nursing practice.* Menlo Park, CA: Addison-Wesley Publishing.

Benner, P., Tanner, C., & Chelsa, C. (2009). *Expertise in nursing practice: Caring, clinical judgment, and ethics* (2nd ed.). New York: Springer Publishing.

Curry, L. (1983). *An organization of learning styles theories and constructs.* Paper presented at the American Educational Research Association Annual Meeting, Montreal, Canada. Retrieved from http://eric.ed.gov/PDFS/ED235185.pdf

Curry, L. (1987). *Integrating concepts of cognitive or learning style: A review with attention to psychometric standards.* Ottawa, ON: Canadian College of Health Service Executives.

Dreyfus, H. L., & Dreyfus, S. E. (2009). The relationship of theory and practice in the acquisition of skill. In P. Benner, C. Tanner, & C. Chelsa (Eds.), *Expertise in nursing practice: Caring, clinical judgment, and ethics* (2nd ed.) (pp. 1-24). New York: Springer Publishing.

Dreyfus, S. E., & Dreyfus, H. L. (1980). *A five-stage model of the mental activities involved in directed skill acquisition.* Berkeley, CA: University of California Operations Research Center. Retrieved from http://www.dtic.mil/cgi-bin/GetTRDoc?Location=U2&doc=GetTRDoc.pdf&AD=ADA084551

Dunn, R., & Dunn, K. (1978). *Teaching students through their individual learning styles: A practical approach.* Reston, VA: National Association of Secondary School Principals.

Gregorc, A. F. (1979). Learning/teaching styles: Their nature and effects. In J. Keefe (Ed.), *Student learning styles: Diagnosing and prescribing programs* (pp. 19-26). Reston, VA: National Association of Secondary School Principals.

Gregorc, A. F. (1982). *An adult's guide to style*. Maynard, MA: Gabriel Systems.

Gregorc, A. F. (1984). Style as a symptom: A phenomenological perspective. *Theory into Practice, 23*(1), 51-55.

Holton, E. F., Swanson, R. A., & Naquin, S. S. (2001). Andragogy in practice: Clarifying the andragogical model of adult learning. *Performance Improvement Quarterly, 14*(1), 118-143.

Jonassen, D. H., & Grabowski, B. L. (1993). *Handbook of individual differences, learning, and instruction.* Hillsdale, NJ: Lawrence Erlbaum Associates.

Knowles, M. (1973). *The adult learner: A neglected species.* Houston, TX: Gulf Publishing Company.

Knowles, M. (1984). *The adult learner: A neglected species* (3rd ed.). Houston, TX: Gulf Publishing Company.

Knowles, M. (1987). Adult learning. In R. Craig (Ed.), *Training and development handbook* (pp. 168-179). New York: McGraw-Hill.

Knowles, M., Holton III, E., & Swanson, R. (1998). *The adult learner: The definitive classic in adult education and human resource development* (5th ed.). Houston, TX: Gulf Publishing.

Knowles, M., Holton III, E., & Swanson, R. (2005). *The adult learner: The definitive classic in adult education and human resource development* (6th ed.). Burlington, MA: Elsevier.

Kolb, D. A. (1984). *Experiential learning: Experience the source of learning and development.* Englewood Cliffs, NJ: Prentice Hall.

Kolb, D. A. (1999). *Learning style inventory.* Boston, MA: Hay McBer.

Lieb, S. (1991, Fall). Principles of adult learning. *Vision.* Retrieved from http://honolulu.hawaii.edu/intranet/committees/FacDevCom/guidebk/teachtip/adults-2.htm

Lore, A. (1981). *Effective therapeutic communications.* Bourne, MD: Robert J. Brady Co.

Maslow, A. H. (1954). *Motivation and personality.* New York: Harper.

Maslow, A. H. (1971). *The farther reaches of human nature.* New York: The Viking Press.

Maslow, A. H., & Lowery, R. (Eds.). (1998). *Toward a psychology of being* (3rd ed.). New York: John Wiley & Sons.

Merriam, S. B., & Caffarella, R. S. (1999). *Learning in adulthood: A comprehensive guide.* San Francisco, CA: Jossey-Bass.

Mezirow, J. (1991). *Transformative dimensions of adult learning.* San Francisco, CA: Jossey-Bass.

Mezirow, J. (1997). Transformative learning: Theory to practice. *New Directions for Adult and Continuing Education, 74,* 5-12.

Myers, I. B., & McCaulley, M. H. (1985). *Manual: A guide to the development and use of the Myers-Briggs Type Indicator.* Palo Alto, CA: Consulting Psychologists Press.

Smith, J. (2002). Learning styles: Fashion fad or lever for change? The application of learning style theory to inclusive curriculum delivery. *Innovations in Education and Teaching International, 39*(10), 63-70.

Sternberg, R. J. (1997). *Thinking styles.* New York: Cambridge University Press.

Witkin, H. A., Oltman, P. K., Raskin, E., & Karp, S. A. (1971). *A manual for the embedded figures tests.* Palo Alto, CA: Consulting Psychologists Press.

Zemke, R., & Zemke, S. (1995, June). Adult learning: What do we know for sure? *Training, 32*(6), 31-40.

**Preceptor Development Plan
Learning Theories and Styles**

Think about the learning theories and styles described in this chapter. How do you learn best?

Name:

How I learn best:

Note: This form and other resources are available at www.RNPreceptor.com.

"Education is the kindling of the flame, not the filling of the vessel."

–Socrates

Precepting Strategies

Beth Tamplet Ulrich, EdD, RN, FACHE, FAAN

3

As you begin your precepting role, you need to understand the basic strategies used in precepting. Clarifying the preceptor role is a first step, followed by understanding precepting models, sharing information, engaging others, conducting a preceptee learner assessment, helping the preceptee manage transitions, using clinical teaching strategies, and finally, ending the preceptor-preceptee relationship. This chapter provides an overview of these strategies to get you started in your new role.

Getting Started

At the outset (or, better yet, before you decide to accept the preceptor role), you need to have a detailed conversation with your manager about your role as a preceptor. At a minimum, you should discuss:

- The outcomes your manager expects from you as a preceptor and from preceptees.

- The preceptor role requirements

- The support available for you and your preceptees

- The amount of time that will be dedicated to the preceptor and preceptee roles

- The priority of your precepting role with your other duties

Statements such as the following are red flags to potential future role conflict issues: "Just teach her what you know." "You're very efficient. You can just work it in with your patient care, can't you?"

OBJECTIVES

- Understand basic precepting strategies

- Know how to begin a preceptor-preceptee relationship

- Use teaching strategies in the preceptor role

"You're an experienced nurse. You'll figure it out." It is much easier and much less frustrating to address these issues before you start precepting. Some sample detailed questions are shown in Table 3.1. In organizations with structured preceptorships, many of the topics will have already been addressed and decisions made.

Table 3.1   Role Clarification

Expected Outcomes

- At what level of practice do you expect the preceptee to be at the end of the preceptorship?
- What specific competencies do you expect the preceptee to have at the end of the preceptorship?

Preceptor Role Requirements

- What are your expectations of me?
- Are there classes I need to take?
- Are there continuing education requirements?
- Will I need to liaison with anyone (i.e., nursing school faculty for student nurses)?

Support Available for the Preceptor and Preceptee

- What initial preparation will I get for the preceptor role? Will additional education be available in the future?
- Who is available for me as resources? Will I have an experienced preceptor to precept me in my preceptor role?
- What information resources are available to me and my preceptee?
- If the preceptee is a new graduate, do we have a structured RN residency or transition to practice program in place? Will there be training for me?

Time Dedicated to the Preceptor and Preceptee Roles

- How much of my time will be dedicated to the preceptor role for each type of preceptee (i.e., new graduate nurse, new hire experienced nurse, experienced nurse new to our specialty)?
- How much preceptee time will be dedicated to the preceptee role for each type of preceptee (i.e., new graduate nurse, new hire experienced nurse, experienced nurse new to our specialty)?
- What part of my hours and my preceptee's hours will be counted in staffing?

Priority of the Precepting Role With Other Duties

- Except for emergencies, will I be pulled to staff other shifts or units when I'm in my preceptor role? If yes, will someone take my place with my preceptee?

Precepting Models

In the initial use of precepting in nursing (mid 1970s), a preceptor was assigned to a preceptee, but too often, the preceptor and the preceptee were not always on the same shifts, or the preceptor got pulled away during the shift. In the best cases, another preceptor was assigned to the preceptee, but often preceptees were left on their own until their next shift with their preceptor. Such unplanned changes in preceptors often resulted in "lost shifts" and/or confusion for the preceptee and frustration for the preceptors. Preceptor inconsistency appeared to be a particular problem for new graduate nurse preceptees, who did not yet have a foundation of clinical experience on which to rely. As new graduate residencies were developed, those developing the residencies began to address the preceptor issues.

Single Preceptor Model

In the single preceptor model, the preceptee is assigned one preceptor. The advantage of the single preceptor model is that, in theory, it provides for continuity, especially if a commitment to schedule the preceptor and preceptee on the same shifts exists. The problem is maintaining that continuity in the real world of hospital staffing. Because of the potential lack of matching preceptor and preceptee shifts, the single preceptor model might well be the best model for use with preceptees who are experienced nurses new to the organization or in new specialties or roles, but can be less advantageous for novice nurses who do not yet have a foundation of experience.

Team Preceptor Model

The team preceptor model has been used most often with new graduate nurses. Versant, an early leader in the development of structured RN residencies, created a team preceptor model in response to identified problems using traditional preceptor approaches with new graduate nurses. Versant began its RN residency in 1999, assigning a preceptor and an alternate preceptor for each preceptee (Beecroft, Hernandez, & Reid, 2008). All of the preceptors were expert nurses.

After several cohorts of residents, it became apparent that, despite the attempts to provide more consistency with preceptors, improvements in the preceptor program were needed. Too often, if the primary and alternate preceptors were unavailable, any available nurse was substituted. In addition, it was clear that the same nurses were being called on over and over to precept, and the potential for burnout was high (Beecroft et al., 2008).

Also, using only expert nurses as preceptors of new graduates was frustrating for everyone. The expert nurses, who were at an intuitive level of practice, found it hard to break down their practice to the 1-2-3, A-B-C steps that new graduate nurses needed to learn at the novice level. In turn, the new graduate nurses were not progressing as quickly as they wanted to when they got caught in preceptor musical chairs. Versant moved to a team precepting model, which has become the practice standard of the Versant RN Residency (Ulrich et al., 2010).

In the team preceptor model, a team of preceptors at various levels of competence work together to precept the new graduate nurse. The new graduate's first preceptor is a newly competent nurse who has an experience level closer to that of the new graduate. The newly competent nurse as preceptor remembers well what it was like to be a new graduate nurse and understands how to work with the recent graduate. The use of newly competent nurses as preceptors also provides an opportunity for them to engage in the work of the organization in a new way and recognizes their professional development and potential.

As the new graduate nurse gains knowledge and expertise, a preceptor with more clinical experience takes over the preceptor responsibility, and finally, in the last part of the immersion period of the Versant RN Residency, an expert nurse preceptor works with the new graduate nurse. Critical components of this team preceptor model are transparency and accountability as well as a communication and documentation system that allows easy access by all involved to preceptee-related information (i.e., competency validation, notes on strengths, and areas for improvement).

Preceptee Cohorts or One at a Time?

Preceptees can be singles or grouped in cohorts. Cohorts have been used successfully for new graduate nurses and specialty nurse education. The single preceptee versus cohort approach has implications for preceptors.

When a preceptee is a single, all of the responsibility falls to the preceptor. This might not be a problem if the preceptee is an experienced nurse in a new job or a new role. Precepting in these situations generally requires less structure and less direct observation by the preceptor. Precepting a single new graduate or a single nurse in a new specialty can be labor-intensive and emotionally intensive for the preceptor.

Cohorts often have more committed resources and structure. For example, in a cohort of nurses learning neonatal intensive care as a new specialty, classes or learning with human patient simulators can occur as a group, with objectives established for what each preceptee is to accomplish prior to the next session. Cohorts also provide the opportunity for group meetings, such as debriefing sessions with new graduates. And for preceptors, cohorts provide the potential of preceptors for the cohort supporting each other, sharing ideas and strategies, and problem-solving as a group.

Sharing Information

Regardless of the preceptorship model—one preceptor or a team of preceptors, single preceptees or cohorts—key components to the success of precepting are communication, transparency, and accountability among all those involved: the preceptee, preceptor(s), manager, charge nurse, etc. These components mimic those required for successful patient handoffs.

Riesenberg, Leitzsch, and Cunningham (2010), in an extensive nursing literature review, found eight major categories of barriers to effective patient handoffs.

1. Communication barriers were the most frequent (general communication problems, social and hierarchical problems, cultural issues)

2. Problems associated with standardization (lack of standardization)

3. Equipment issues (limitations associated with the communication medium)

4. Environmental issues (interruptions, distractions)

5. A lack of or misuse of time (time constraints)

6. Difficulties related to complexity of cases or a high caseload (too many patients, more complex handoffs)

7. A lack of training or education (inadequate or no training)

8. Human factors (too few nurses, sensory and information overload)

All of these barriers can also apply to preceptee handoffs. Just as inadequate patient handoffs can increase costs, misuse resources, and result in poorer patient outcomes, so too can inadequate preceptee handoffs increase costs, misuse resources, and result in poorer preceptee outcomes.

Riesenberg and colleagues (2010) also identified strategies for effective patient handoffs. These strategies, too, can also be applied to preceptee handoffs.

- Communication skills (general communication, preparation, transfer of responsibility, language)

- Standardization strategies (standardize the process, use interactive questioning during face-to-face communication, monitor the process)

- Technologic solutions (use an electronic handoff system)

- Environmental strategies (limit interruptions and distractions)

- Training and education (provide adequate refresher training or education)

- Staff involvement (involve staff)

- Leadership (have consistent expectations for compliance)

Preceptors need access to a system of documentation and communication with everyone involved with the preceptee. Characteristics of such a system include easy access, easy use, and confidentiality as indicated. For example, preceptors need to see at a glance which competencies have been validated and which have not. If charge nurses also have access to this information, they can take it into consideration when making assignments or when opportunities come up to do certain procedures. If the manager can see the information on the preceptee, he or she will know the preceptee's progress or lack of progress and can support the preceptor's efforts.

It Takes a Village

Bringing someone new into a position or role truly does take a village. Though the preceptor takes the lead and is the "go-to" person for the preceptee, the preceptor needs the support of others to be successful. Engaging others can help you as the preceptor and can give the preceptee opportunities to form new relationships. Colleagues can be alert to practice opportunities that will help develop the preceptee's competence. Physicians, pharmacists, social workers, and other health professionals can assist in teaching the preceptee. All can be supportive of the preceptee's need to learn and be socialized into the organization and the unit.

Establishing the Preceptor-Preceptee Relationship

It is relatively rare for any matching to be done between preceptors and preceptees, so establishing a relationship with the preceptee is pretty much starting from scratch. If possible, spend some one-on-one time with the preceptee as soon as possible. Go on a break or have lunch together. Spend a little time just getting to know each other.

Role clarification comes next. Discuss your role and the preceptee's role. What are you each responsible for? If the preceptee will be participating in a structured program such as a new graduate residency or specialty nursing education, discuss how the preceptorship fits into the program.

Begin to build trust. Bracey (2002) has developed a five-step trust-building model.

1. Be transparent (open, easily readable, and vulnerable)

2. Be responsive (give honest feedback respectfully, spontaneously, and non-judgmentally)

3. Use caring (whatever is said or done comes from the heart; behavior is compassionate, affirming, and understanding)

4. Be sincere (congruent, integral, accountable, actions are consistent with words)

5. Be trustworthy (honest, honor your word, manage by agreements)

Remember that trust is a two-way street. As the preceptor, you hold the power in the relationship (whether you like to think of it that way or not, it is reality), and you must be especially vigilant where trust is concerned.

You also need to discuss ground rules and relationship agreements at the beginning. One example is establishing a way to communicate in critical or unsafe situations. For example, you and the preceptee are in a patient's room, and you see the preceptee doing something incorrectly. You don't want to call her out on it in a way that might alarm the patient, but you need to step in. One suggestion is to agree on a word or phrase that you can say in those situations so the preceptee knows that you need to take over (Modic & Schoessler, 2008). Another example would be to discuss that there might be times in emergency situations when you must act and cannot take the time to teach, and when you need the preceptee to act quickly and not expect explanations until later. Again, you and the preceptee can agree on a code word or phrase that, in essence, means "do what I say and do it now—we'll talk about it later." The agreement should include a commitment to debrief after the emergency is over.

Another example of a ground rule would be that the preceptee commits to let you know when she is unsure of what you mean or doesn't understand something. One of my colleagues, Dr. Sean Early, taught me a technique to use while teaching classes. He stacks three cups in front of each attendee—a green cup, a yellow cup, and a red cup. He then tells the attendees that the top cup is their signal to him and the rest of the group of where they are in understanding what is being discussed. The green cup means "I'm with you. Keep going." The yellow cup means "I need clarification" or "I may be getting lost." It is a signal for the presenter to stop and offer assistance, clarification, etc., and to keep doing that until the green cup is put back on top. The red cup means "Stop right now; you've lost me," and is the indicator that the presenter needs to stop immediately and help the attendee. The interesting things about this process are how quickly you, as the presenter, can have an almost Pavlovian response to the cup colors and how even the shyest attendees, who might have never spoken up, will use the cups to communicate their needs. You can't use cups in clinical teaching, but you can develop an equivalent way for preceptees to communicate their needs.

Preceptee Learner Assessment

You need to have a starting point for the precepting experience. You cannot assume that the preceptee has knowledge or expertise based on his or her educational degree or past experience. Learner assessment starts with conversations. Case studies, simulation scenarios, and online testing can be used to assess competencies. Prompts such as "Tell me how you would handle XYZ" can be enlightening. If preceptees balk at the need for you to do a preliminary assessment or for them to demonstrate knowledge and/or competency, explain that your obligation is first and foremost to make sure that the patients receive safe, quality care and that the only way you can let the preceptees care for patients is if you know their level of competence.

Managing Transitions

Preceptees are transitioning into a new world, and that new world might mean transitioning from student to professional nurse, into a new role or specialty, or into a new organization. William Bridges (1991, p. 3) says, "It's not the changes that do you in, it's the transitions. Change is not the same as transition. Change is situational: the new site, the new boss, the new team roles, the new policy. Transition is the psychological process people go through to come to terms with the new situation. Change is external, transition is internal." Or as Marilyn Ferguson (as cited in Bridges, 1991), a futurist, describes it, "It's not so much that we're afraid of change or so in love with the old ways, but it's that place in between that we fear . . . It's like being between trapezes. It's Linus when his blanket is in the dryer. There's nothing to hold onto" (p. 34).

As the preceptor, you must be attuned to the effect that being in a state of transition can have on preceptees. This is especially true with new graduate nurses who are going through personal and professional transition. They're paying rent. They no longer have every weekend off. There's no summer vacation. They have to work 12-hour days. They're learning to balance life and work. If you're precepting new managers, the transition might be particularly hard if they've been promoted from within and they now supervise people who were their peers last week. Sometimes a simple "How's it going?" is enough to show that you have an understanding of how hard transitions can be and that you are available to help if needed. Another strategy is to verbally paint preceptees a mental picture of what it will look like in their new world when the transition is done. Bridges (1991) suggests reinforcing the new beginning by being consistent, ensuring quick successes, symbolizing the new identity, and celebrating success.

Clinical Teaching Strategies

Preceptors can use a number of teaching strategies. Four of the most common are the strengths-based approach, the five-step microskills model of clinical teaching, debriefing, and reflective practice.

Strengths-Based Approach

The strengths-based approach, according to Saleebey (2002), emphasizes discovering, affirming, and enhancing the capabilities, interests, knowledge, resources, and goals of individuals. For many preceptees, the preceptor will have to begin the strengths-based approach by explaining it to the preceptees. Preceptees whose past experiences have been predominantly with deficit-based approaches and one-way, teacher-directed communication have to adjust to not hearing mainly what they've done wrong and generally "waiting for the other shoe to drop" in communications. Using the strengths-based approach, the preceptor facilitates discovery and clinical reflection and creates a learning environment that is based on mutuality and building on strengths. Cederbaum and Klusaritz (2009) identify several tenets of the strengths-based approach: self-determination, empowerment, mutuality, collaboration, reflection on change, community membership, and regeneration.

Cederbaum and Klusaritz (2009) also offer some practical suggestions on using the strengths-based approach with students that we have adapted for use in all precepting endeavors:

- Use a learning contract—The learning contract emphasizes the mutual process between preceptors and preceptees and delineates roles and responsibilities of both participants. The contract can be a verbal agreement or a written agreement, as suggested by Cederbaum and Klusaritz (2009).

- Express concerns in a positive manner—The strengths-based approach, in contrast to the often used deficit-based approach, emphasizes identifying and building on existing strengths. It does not mean that deficits and problems are not addressed but, rather, that they and the actions needed are framed in a positive manner.

- See the learning process through preceptees' eyes—Preceptors can use the strengths-based approach to help them understand how preceptees view the clinical situation and the learning environment. Preceptors can work with preceptees to create a plan to address any concerns.

- Create a safe practice environment—The preceptor is responsible for assuring that preceptees have a safe environment in which to learn, including physical and mental safety.

- Practice tolerance—Being a preceptor isn't easy. Preceptees will sometimes not share your beliefs, skills, views, etc. They often (hopefully) have a lot of questions, and their pace of both thought and action is generally not as fast as the preceptor's pace. Being a preceptor includes accepting that your way is not the only way, and preceptors can often learn from their preceptees.

- Examining teaching style—Reflecting on your own teaching style and being open to new ideas and strategies enhance your effectiveness as a preceptor.

Ken Blanchard and Spencer Johnson (1981), in their long-acclaimed book, *The One Minute Manager*, put it very simply: "Help people reach their full potential. Catch them doing something right" (p. 39). Details on their suggestions for one-minute praising are found in Table 3.2.

Table 3.2   One-Minute Praising
• Tell people up-front that you are going to let them know how they are doing.
• Praise people immediately.
• Tell people what they did right—be specific.
• Tell people how good you feel about what they did right and how it helps the organization and the other people who work there.
• Stop for a moment of silence to let them "feel" how good you feel.
• Encourage them to do more of the same.
• Shake hands or touch people in a way that makes it clear that you support their success in the organization.

Source: Blanchard & Johnson, 1981, p. 44.

One other suggestion is what Michael LeBoeuf (1985) calls the greatest management principle in the world—"The things that get rewarded get done." He goes on to say, "The greatest single obstacle to the success of today's organizations is the giant mismatch between the behavior we need and the behavior we reward" (p. 9). Rewards come in many forms, and you have to be careful not to unintentionally reward behavior that you don't want. For example, if you pay a lot of attention and express concern when your preceptee is whiny and not so much attention and concern when the preceptee is acting more professional, and if the preceptee likes to receive your attention and concern, what behavior do you think will be repeated most? With a strengths-based approach, you need to make sure that strengths, and building on strengths, are what gets rewarded.

Microskills Model

Neher and colleagues (1992) created the five-step microskills model of clinical teaching to provide efficient and effective teaching in the clinical setting for family practice students and residents. More recently, this model has been referred to as the one-minute preceptor (Neher & Stevens, 2003), although in practice the model generally takes more than one minute. The five steps of the model are as follows:

1. Get a commitment to a diagnosis and/or course of action by engaging the student in an interactive learning experience.

2. Probe for supporting evidence; find out how the decision was made.

3. Teach general rules; discuss how what was learned in this experience can be applied more generally.

4. Reinforce what was done right; be specific.

5. Correct mistakes and/or discuss common mistakes to avoid.

The one-minute preceptor model has also been used in nursing with positive results. Bott, Mohide, and Lawlor (2011), after reviewing the model and doing a literature review, modified the model to better fit nursing and renamed it the five minute preceptor, to better reflect the actual time for using the model. The steps of the five minute preceptor model are as follows (Bott et al., 2011):

1. Get the student to take a stand—This statement allows for the broader options and situations that the nurse might be experiencing beyond diagnoses and courses of action in the first step of the one-minute preceptor model. In this step, the preceptor would use general questions or comments to help the student/preceptee work through his or her thought process.

2. Probe for supporting evidence—In this second step, the preceptor "asks clearly framed, higher order questions to elicit evidence or rationale" (Bott et al., 2011, p. 38) and to determine how the preceptee decided on the decision in step one. This action provides the opportunity for the preceptor to identify any preceptee learning needs or knowledge gaps.

3. Teach general rules—Having done the previous two steps, the preceptor has a wonderful opportunity to extend the preceptee's knowledge and learning in the current specific situation to more general situations.

4. Reinforce the positives—In this step, the preceptor "provides positive feedback with rationale or explanations that reinforce the student's strengths and competencies (knowledge, skills, and/or attitudes), so that positives can be applied reliably in future situations" (Bott et al., 2011, p. 39). Feedback should be very specific.

5. Correct errors or misinterpretations—The preceptor provides constructive feedback and additional relevant information and discusses with the preceptee how to apply this information in the future.

Bott and colleagues note that in their analysis of the five minute preceptor model, they recognized a strong parallel between the model and the experiential learning process described by Kolb (1984).

Parrott and colleagues (2006), after reviewing the research on the one-minute preceptor model, summarized the factors that had been found to contribute to the success of the model:

- The clinical teacher's ability to correctly diagnose the patient's problem

- The clinical teacher's confidence in evaluating the learner

- The clinical teacher's ability to encourage the learner to do independent learning and outside reading

- The quality of feedback that clinical teachers give to learners (high order feedback is better)

- The frequency with which clinical teachers give feedback to learners (more is better)

Debriefing

To achieve maximum learning, you need to have time to debrief after clinical experiences to review the experience in a systematic and purposeful way. Warrick and colleagues (1979) note that debriefing is designed to synergize, strengthen, and transfer learning, but also that it is often the most overlooked part of the experiential learning process. They have found that for meaningful and transferable learning to occur, there should be an opportunity for learners to reflect on their experience, receive specific behavioral feedback, integrate observation and feedback within conceptual frameworks, and create mechanisms for transferring learning to other situations. This coincides with the learning cycle described by Kolb (1984) of the concrete experience, reflective observation, abstract conceptualization, and active experimentation (see Chapter 2 for additional information).

The objectives for debriefing include:

- Identify and discuss what occurred from the perspectives of the preceptee and the preceptor (clinical and behavioral aspects).

- Transfer of knowledge—Link the experience to evidence, theory, practice guidelines, and skill-building specific to this experience. Reinforce teaching points.

- Answer the preceptee's questions.

- Identify potential resources.

- Enhance critical thinking, clinical reasoning, and clinical judgment skills.
- Summarize the key points of the experience and what was learned.

Debriefing is best done as close in time to the event as possible to better capture recall of events, thinking, and feelings. In the clinical setting, this might mean taking time during the shift to do a short debriefing for critical events and a longer debriefing at the end of the shift that covers the experiences of the day. This is especially the case for new graduates who are experiencing major events for the first time, such as the death of a patient, an ethics issue, or a code. All debriefings—short or long—need to occur in an environment in which the preceptee feels safe.

The preceptor's ability to communicate is a critical factor in the success of debriefing. Listening attentively to what preceptees say and being able to articulate and summarize succinctly what occurred and what is to be learned are both important elements. Detailed information on communication can be found in Chapter 6.

Rudolph and colleagues (2006) discuss the two extremes of debriefing, judgmental and nonjudgmental, and find both lacking. The judgmental approach "places truth solely in the possession of the instructor, error in the hands of the trainee, and presumes that there is an essential failure in the thinking or actions of the trainee" (p. 51). They further note that "a judgmental approach to debriefing, especially one that includes harsh criticism, can have serious costs: humiliation, dampened motivation, reluctance to raise questions about later areas of confusion, or exit of talented trainees from the specialty or clinical practice altogether" (p. 51).

On the other hand, preceptors using the nonjudgmental approach might employ protective social strategies (i.e., sugarcoating, surrounding the negative with more positives) and not address critical issues, thereby inadvertently implying that what is not discussed is unimportant or that mistakes should not be talked about.

Rudolph et al. (2006) propose another option—debriefing with good judgment. This approach "values the expert opinion of the instructors, while at the same time valuing the unique perspective of the trainees. The idea is to learn what participant frames drive their behaviors so that both their 'failures' and successes can be understood as an ingenious, inevitable and logical solution to the problem as perceived within their frames" (p. 52). The debriefing with good judgment approach focuses on creating a context for adult learners to learn important lessons that can help them move toward key objectives and includes the learner's meaning-making systems and the sharing of insights by the instructor to initiate dialog. Errors are openly discussed, so they can be a source of learning.

Rudolph and colleagues (2006) suggest using an advocacy-inquiry approach, with advocacy being an assertion, observation, or statement, and inquiry being a question. After noticing a result and observing what actions led to the result, the instructor uses advocacy-inquiry to discover the frames or context that guided the learner's actions. This approach helps preceptees articulate their thinking and reasoning and gives preceptors the opportunity to help preceptees identify gaps or errors and learn from the experience.

Reflective Practice

Dewey (1933, p. 3) defines reflection as "the turning over of a subject in the mind and giving it serious and consecutive consideration." *Reflective practice* is a term coined by Schoen (1983) to describe examining the knowledge base, values, and assumptions that drive your professional practice. Schoen discusses two types of reflection—reflection in practice or reflection in action, which occurs during an action or practice, and reflection on practice or reflection on action, which occurs after.

Johns (1994) created a model of structured reflection. It includes a description of the reflection experience (i.e., What was I trying to achieve? Why did I act as I did? What were the consequences? How did I feel? How did others feel? How do I know how others felt?); influencing factors (internal and external); and learning (What were other options? What would be the consequences of those options? How has the experience changed my way of knowing?). These cues can be used to assist individuals in reflective thinking.

Reflective learning is important for both preceptors and preceptees. Scanlan and Chernomas (1997) say that "to teach reflectively, we must be reflective ourselves" (p. 1141). They describe being a reflective teacher as thinking about your teaching, modeling reflective thinking strategies, and using teaching strategies that encourage the learner to be reflective. Not everyone is skilled in self-reflection or comfortable engaging in it. Part of the work of preceptors is to learn to be reflective in their own practice and to encourage and support self-reflection by preceptees.

Ending the Preceptor-Preceptee Relationship

Just as important as how you begin the preceptor-preceptee relationship is how you end it. A final meeting with just you and the preceptee and another meeting with you, the preceptee, and the manager are important for closure and to assure that the preceptee's growth and learning will continue. Closure allows affirmation and action planning, ties things together, and allows and encourages celebration.

In the meeting with you and the preceptee, at a minimum:

- Review the preceptorship, covering the highlights.

- Acknowledge any loose ends or unfinished work, and discuss a plan for completion.

- Recognize the preceptee's growth.

- Acknowledge what you have learned.

- Ask for feedback for the preceptorship as a whole and for you as a preceptor.

- Ask about the preceptee's future plans, and offer to be of help.

At the meeting with the preceptee and the manager:

- Discuss the preceptorship as a whole.

- Recognize the preceptee's growth.

- Discuss any additional work that the preceptee needs to complete and assist in developing a plan for completion.

Last, but not least, celebrate, preferably with the unit as a whole, to acknowledge completion of the preceptorship. Some organizations literally have a "cut the cord" ceremony symbolizing the advancement of the preceptees. Find whatever works in your culture for celebrations to acknowledge the completion of this transition.

Conclusion

The general precepting strategies discussed in this chapter should be considered as you move into the preceptor role and begin preceptor-preceptee relationships. By clarifying your manager's expectations of the preceptor role at the beginning, you will better understand the work you are to do and the conditions under which you are to do the work. Understanding the prevalent preceptorship models will help you know the advantages and disadvantages of each model. Using the strategies for starting, maintaining, and ending a relationship will let you plan the overall preceptorship and assure that both you and your preceptee are successful.

References

Beecroft, P., Hernandez, A. M., & Reid, D. (2008). Team preceptorships: A new approach for precepting new nurses. *Journal for Nurses in Staff Development, 24*(4), 143-148.

Blanchard, K. H., & Johnson, S. (1981). *The one minute manager.* New York, NY: Blanchard Family Partnership.

Bott, G., Mohide, E. A., & Lawlor, Y. (2011). A clinical teaching technique for nurse preceptors: The five minute preceptor. *Journal of Professional Nursing, 27*(1), 35-42.

Bracey, H. (2002). *Building trust: How to get it! How to keep it!* Charleston, SC: Createspace.

Bridges, W. (1991). *Managing transitions: Making the most of change.* Reading, MA: Addison-Wesley Publishing Company.

Cederbaum, J., & Klusaritz, H. A. (2009). Clinical instruction: Using the strengths-based approach with nursing students. *Journal of Nursing Education, 48*(8), 422-428.

Dewey, J. (1933). *How we think.* New York, NY: D. C. Heath.

Johns, C. (1994). Guided reflection. In A. Palmer, B. Burns, & C. Bulman (Eds.), *Reflective practice in nursing.* Oxford: Blackwell Science.

Kolb, D. A. (1984). *Experiential learning: Experience the source of learning and development.* Englewood Cliffs, NJ: Prentice Hall.

LeBoeuf, M. (1985). *The greatest management principle in the world.* New York, NY: G. P. Putnam's Sons.

Modic, M. B., & Schoessler, M. (2008). Preceptorship. *Journal for Nurses in Staff Development, 24*(1), 43-44.

Neher, J. O., Gordon, K. C., Meyer, B., & Stevens, N. (1992). A five-step "microskills" model of clinical teaching. *Journal of the American Board of Family Practice, 5*(4), 419-424.

Neher, J. O., & Stevens, N. (2003). The one-minute preceptor: Shaping the teaching conversation. *Family Medicine, 35*(6), 391-393.

Parrott, S., Dobbie, A., Chumley, H., & Tysinger, J. W. (2006). Evidence-based office teaching—The five-step microskills model of clinical teaching. *Family Medicine, 38*(3), 164-167.

Riesenberg, L.A., Leitzsch, J., & Cunningham, J.M. (2010). Nursing handoffs: A systematic review of the literature. *American Journal of Nursing, 110*(4), 24-34.

Rudolph, J., Simon, R., Dufresne, R., & Raemer, D. (2006). There's no such thing as "nonjudgmental" debriefing: A theory and method of debriefing with good judgment. *Simulation in Healthcare, 1*(1), 49-55.

Saleebey, D. (2002). *The strengths perspective in social work practice* (3rd ed.). Boston: Allyn & Bacon.

Scanlan, J. M., & Chernomas, W. M. (1997). Developing the reflective teacher. *Journal of Advanced Nursing, 25*(6), 1138-1143.

Schoen, D. A. (1983). *The reflective practitioner: How professionals think in action.* New York, NY: Basic Books.

Ulrich, B., Krozek, C., Early, S., Ashlock, C. H., Africa, L. M., & Carman, M. L. (2010). Improving retention, confidence, and competence of new graduate nurses: Results from a 10-year longitudinal database. *Nursing Economic$, 28*(6), 363-376.

Warrick, D. D., Hunsaker, P. L., Cook, C. W., & Altman, S. (1979). Debriefing experiential learning exercises. *Journal of Experiential Learning and Simulation, 1,* 91-100.

Preceptor Development Plan
Precepting Strategies: Preceptor Role Clarification

Clarify the preceptor role with your manager.

Review the precepting strategies described in this chapter. What are your strengths? In which areas do you need to increase your knowledge and expertise? What is your plan for expanding your knowledge and expertise? What resources are available? Who can help you?

Name:	
Manager's Name:	
Expected Outcomes	
At what level of practice do you expect the preceptee to be at the end of the preceptorship?	
What specific competencies do you expect the preceptee to have at the end of the preceptorship?	
Preceptor Role Requirements	
What are your expectations of me?	
Are there classes I need to take?	
Are there continuing education requirements?	
Will I need to liaison with anyone (for example, nursing school faculty for student nurses)?	
Support Available for the Preceptor and the Preceptee	
What initial preparation will I get for the preceptor role?	
Will additional education be available in the future? If so, what?	
Who is available to me as resources?	
Will I have an experienced preceptor to precept me in my preceptor role?	
What information resources are available to me and my preceptee?	
If the preceptee is a new graduate, do we have a structured RN residency or transition to practice program in place? Will there be training for me on that program?	

Time Dedicated to the Preceptor and Preceptee Roles	
How much of my time will be dedicated to the preceptor role for each type of preceptee (for example, new graduate nurse, new hire experienced nurse, experienced nurse new to our specialty)?	
How much preceptee time will be dedicated to the preceptee role for each type of preceptee (for example, new graduate nurse, new hire experienced nurse, experienced nurse new to our specialty)?	
What part of my hours and my preceptee's hours will be counted in staffing?	
Priority of Precepting Role With Other Duties	
Except for emergencies, will I be pulled to staff other shifts or units when I'm in my preceptor role? If yes, will someone take my place with my preceptee?	
Other Items/Issues Discussed	

Note: This form and other resources are available at www.RNPreceptor.com.

Preceptor Development Plan Precepting Strategies			
Name:			
Sharing Information			
Strengths	Needs	Plan	Resources
It Takes a Village—Engaging Others			
Strengths	Needs	Plan	Resources
Establishing the Preceptor-Preceptee Relationship			
Strengths	Needs	Plan	Resources
Preceptee Learner Assessment			
Strengths	Needs	Plan	Resources
Managing Transitions			
Strengths	Needs	Plan	Resources
Clinical Teaching Strategies			
Strengths	Needs	Plan	Resources
Ending the Preceptee-Preceptee Relationship			
Strengths	Needs	Plan	Resources

Note: This form and other resources are available at www.RNPreceptor.com.

"The most important practical lesson that can be given to nurses is to teach them what to observe, how to observe, what symptoms indicate improvement, what the reverse, which are of importance, which are of none, which are evidence of neglect and of what kind of neglect."

–Florence Nightingale

Competence, Critical Thinking, Clinical Judgment and Reasoning, and Confidence

4

Beth Tamplet Ulrich, EdD, RN, FACHE, FAAN

OBJECTIVES

- Understand development of preceptee competence

- Understand critical thinking, clinical reasoning, and clinical judgment and how to help preceptees develop each skill

- Understand the development of preceptee confidence

At the heart of any precepting experience is the development of competence, the development of ability and experiences to effectively utilize the competence (critical thinking, clinical reasoning, and clinical judgment), and the confidence to take action when needed. All must exist for the nurse to practice effectively and safely.

Competence

The American Nurses Association (ANA; 2010) defines a *competency* as "an expected level of performance that integrates knowledge, skills, abilities, and judgment" (p. 12). Knowledge, skills, ability, and judgment are defined as follows (ANA, 2010, pp. 12-13):

- Knowledge encompasses thinking, understanding of science and humanities, professional standards of practice, and insights gained from context, practical experiences, personal capabilities, and leadership performance.

- Skills include psychomotor, communication, interpersonal, and diagnostic skills.

- Ability is the capacity to act effectively. It requires listening, integrity, knowledge of one's strengths and weaknesses, positive self-regard, emotional intelligence, and openness to feedback.

- Judgment includes critical thinking, problem solving, ethical reasoning, and decision-making.

The purposes of ensuring the competence of nurses are protecting the public (the primary purpose), advancing the profession, and ensuring the integrity of the profession (ANA, 2003, 2008). Requirements for competence and competency assessment have been established by national nursing and nursing specialty organizations, state boards of nursing, credentialing boards, and statutory and regulatory agencies. The presence (or absence) of competency can also be a legal issue.

ANA Position Statement on Professional Role Competence

The public has a right to expect registered nurses to demonstrate professional competence throughout their careers. ANA believes the registered nurse is individually responsible and accountable for maintaining professional competence. The ANA further believes that it is the nursing profession's responsibility to shape and guide any process for assuring nurse competence. Regulatory agencies define minimal standards for regulation of practice to protect the public. The employer is responsible and accountable to provide an environment conducive to competent practice. Assurance of competence is the shared responsibility of the profession, individual nurses, professional organizations, credentialing and certification entities, regulatory agencies, employers, and other stakeholders.

Source: ANA, 2008

Competence is not about checking items off a list. In fact, the frequent use of terms such as "competency checklist" and "checking off preceptees" devalues the work required to develop and maintain competence and makes the process of validating competence sound as if it requires little thought—that it is merely an inconsequential nuisance and a documentation chore to be completed as quickly as possible. Nothing could be further from the truth. The validation of competence is one of the most critical elements to assure safe, high quality patient care and competent role performance.

Conscious Competence Learning

The concept of conscious competence learning is a description of how individuals learn new competencies. Though it is unclear who originated the much-used levels of the conscious competence model (some authors cite Confucius, Socrates, and even an oriental proverb; others cite more recent sources), the concept serves to remind us that learning a competence happens in stages. The stages of the concept are as follows:

- Unconscious incompetence—You don't know what you don't know. This stage is especially dangerous with novices.

- Conscious incompetence—You know you don't know.

- Conscious competence—You know that you know it.

- Unconscious competence—You know it so well, you don't think about it.

- Reflective competence—A fifth level suggested by some for knowing when you've reached unconscious competence and analyzing and being able to articulate how you got there well enough to teach someone else to reach that level. This level is particularly important for preceptors to attain.

This concept supports adult learning theory concerning learner readiness in the recognition that individuals develop competence only after they recognize the relevance of their own incompetence.

Competency Outcomes and Performance Assessment (COPA) Model

Lenburg (1999) developed the Competency Outcomes and Performance Assessment (COPA) model. She describes it as "a holistic but focused model that requires the integration of practice-based outcomes, interactive learning methods, and performance assessment of competencies" (the COPA model, 2nd para.).

The basic framework of the model consists of four guiding questions (Lenburg, 1999):

1. What are the essential competencies and outcomes for contemporary practice? Identifying the required competencies and wording them as practice-based competency outcomes.

2. What are the indicators that define those competencies? Only the behaviors, actions, and responses mandatory for the practice of each competency.

3. What are the most effective ways to learn those competencies?

4. What are the most effective ways to document that learners and/or practitioners have achieved the required competencies? Need to develop a systematic and comprehensive plan for outcomes assessment.

Eight core practice competency categories define practice in the COPA model (Lenburg, 1999):

1. Assessment and intervention skills

2. Communication skills

3. Critical thinking skills

4. Human caring and relationship skills

5. Management skills

6. Leadership skills

7. Teaching skills

8. Knowledge integration skills

In the COPA model, learner performance is assessed against a predetermined standard after the learning and practice have occurred. Lenburg (1999) notes how important it is to separate these activities—assessing versus learning/practicing—to keep the focus of each clear. The learner is then better able to concentrate on learning, and the preceptor can concentrate on teaching and coaching during the learning and practice periods, rather than both trying to split their attention and their purposes between learning and assessing and, perhaps, one not always knowing the focus of the other.

Lenburg (1999) has found that assessments are most effective when they are designed and implemented based on 10 basic concepts, including examination, dimensions of practice, critical elements, objectivity, sampling, acceptability, comparability, consistency, flexibility, and systematized conditions.

Competence Development

Seeking to better understand the development of competency, the National Council of State Boards of Nursing (NCSBN) completed a qualitative longitudinal (5-year) study of a national sample of nurses from 2002-2008 (Kearney & Kenward, 2010). By the end of the fifth year, nurses had identified and demonstrated five characteristics of competence:

- Juggling complex patients and assignments efficiently
- Intervening for subtle shifts in patients' conditions or families' responses
- Interpersonal skills of calm, compassion, generosity, and authority
- Seeing the big picture and knowing how to work the system
- An attitude of dedicated curiosity and commitment to lifelong learning

Participants described how competence developed and changed over time. Of interest also was how the development of competency affected their career plans and job satisfaction. Kearny and Kenward (2010) note:

> Those who continued to feel insecure in their ability to efficiently
> identify and respond to important downturns in patients' conditions
> in a high acuity environment, who continually felt beaten down
> in their attempts to get resources and help for patients from fellow
> nurses, and/or who believed physicians did not listen to them or
> respect them appeared most likely to change jobs to less complex or
> less acute settings or to leave nursing. (p. 13)

This study clearly has implications for preceptors. Nurses' career decisions and job satisfaction are both affected by how well they develop competence, especially for less experienced nurses.

Critical Thinking

Critical thinking is a much-used term in nursing in the last 20 years, but a term that gets used loosely and often without definition. Alfaro-LeFevre (1999) notes, "Critical thinking is the key to resolving problems. Nurses who don't think critically become part of the problem" (p. 4). The difference, she says, between thinking and critical thinking is control and purpose. "Thinking is basically any mental activity—it can be aimless and uncontrolled. On the other hand, critical thinking is controlled and purposeful and focuses on using well-reasoned strategies to achieve desired results" (p. 7). Jackson (2006, p. 4) notes that three themes are found within all definitions of critical thinking: "the importance of a good foundation of knowledge, including formal and informal logic; the willingness to ask questions; and the ability to recognize new answers, even when they are not the norm and not in agreement with pre-existing attitudes."

Critical Thinking—A Philosophical Perspective

The American Philosophical Association in 1990 conducted a Delphi study of an expert panel to define critical thinking and to identify and describe the core skills and dispositions of critical thinking. The expert panel, led by Peter Facione (1990), defined critical thinking to be a pervasive and deliberate human phenomenon that is the "purposeful, self-regulatory judgment which results in interpretation, analysis, evaluation, and inference, as well as explanation of the evidential, conceptual, methodological, criteriological, or contextual considerations upon which that judgment is based" (p. 2). The core skills and sub-skills identified by the expert panel are shown in Table 4.1.

According to the American Philosophical Association Delphi Study, the affective dispositions of critical thinking (approaches to life and living) include:

- Inquisitiveness with regard to a wide range of issues

- Concern to become and remain generally well-informed

- Alertness to opportunities to use critical thinking

- Trust in the processes of reasoned inquiry

- Self-confidence in one's own ability to reason

- Open-mindedness regarding divergent world views

- Flexibility in considering alternatives and opinions

- Understanding of the opinions of other people

- Fair-mindedness in appraising reasoning

- Honesty in facing one's own biases, prejudices, stereotypes, and egocentric or sociocentric tendencies

- Prudence in suspending, making, or altering judgments

- Willingness to reconsider and revise views where honest reflection suggests that change is warranted (Facione, 2011)

Table 4.1   Core Critical Thinking Skills and Sub-skills

INTERPRETATION: To comprehend and express the meaning or significance of a wide variety of experiences, situations, data, events, judgments, conventions, beliefs, rules, procedures, or criteria.

Sub-skills: Categorization, decoding significance, clarifying meaning

ANALYSIS: To identify the intended and actual inferential relationships among statements, questions, concepts, descriptions, or other forms of representation intended to express beliefs, judgments, experiences, reasons, information, or opinions.

Sub-skills: Examining ideas, detecting arguments, analyzing arguments

EVALUATION: To assess the credibility of statements or other representations which are accounts or descriptions of a person's perception, experience, situation, judgment, belief, or opinion; and to assess the logical strength of the actual or intended inferential relationships among statements, descriptions, questions, or other forms of representation.

Sub-skills: Assessing claims, assessing arguments

INFERENCE: To identify and secure elements needed to draw reasonable conclusions; to form conjectures and hypotheses; to consider relevant information and to educe the consequences flowing from data, statements, principles, evidence, judgments, beliefs, opinions, concepts, descriptions, questions, or other forms of representation.

Sub-skills: Querying evidence, conjecturing alternatives, drawing conclusions

EXPLANATION: To state the results of one's reasoning; to justify that reasoning in terms of the evidential, conceptual, methodological, criteriological, and contextual considerations upon which one's results were based; and to present one's reasoning in the form of cogent arguments.

Sub-skills: Stating results, justifying procedures, presenting arguments

SELF-REGULATION: Self-consciously to monitor one's cognitive activities, the elements used in those activities, and the results educed, particularly by applying skills in analysis and evaluation to one's own inferential judgments with a view toward questioning, confirming, validating, or correcting either one's reasoning or one's results.

Sub-skills: Self-examination, self-correction

Source: American Philosophical Association, 1990

The dispositions to specific issues, questions, or problems include:

- Clarity in stating the question or concern

- Orderliness in working with complexity

- Diligence in seeking relevant information

- Reasonableness in selecting and applying criteria

- Care in focusing attention on the concern at hand

- Persistence though difficulties are encountered

- Precision to the degree permitted by the subject and the circumstance (Facione, 2011)

Critical Thinking in Nursing

Facione and Facione (1996) suggest that to observe and evaluate critical thinking in nursing knowledge development or clinical decision-making, you need to have the thinking process externalized by being spoken, written, or demonstrated. For preceptors, this means having preceptees externalize their thinking processes. Preceptors must also be able to externalize their own critical thinking to role model critical thinking for preceptees.

Paul, the founder of the Foundation for Critical Thinking, and Heaslip note, "Critical thinking presupposes a certain basic level of intellectual humility (i.e., the willingness to acknowledge the extent of one's own ignorance) and a commitment to think clearly, precisely, and accurately and, in so far as is possible, to act on the basis of genuine knowledge. Genuine knowledge is attained through intellectual effort in figuring out and reasoning about problems one finds in practice" (Paul & Heaslip, 1995, p. 41). Expert nurses, say Paul and Heaslip, "can think through a situation to determine where intuition and ignorance interface with each other" (p. 43).

Building on the work of Facione and the American Philosophical Association Delphi study, Scheffer and Rubenfeld (2000) conducted a Delphi study of international nursing experts (from 27 U.S. states and eight countries) to develop a consensus statement of critical thinking in nursing. The result of the study was a consensus statement and identification of 10 affective components (habits of the mind) and seven cognitive components (skills) of critical thinking in nursing.

> Critical thinking in nursing is an essential component of professional accountability and quality nursing care. Critical thinkers in nursing exhibit these habits of the mind: confidence, contextual perspective, creativity, flexibility, inquisitiveness, intellectual integrity, intuition, open-mindedness, perseverance, and reflection. Critical thinkers in nursing practice the cognitive skills of analyzing, applying standards,

discriminating, information seeking, logical reasoning, predicting and transforming knowledge." (p. 357)

Berkow and colleagues (2011) note that identifying and providing feedback on specific strengths and weaknesses are the first steps to help nurses meaningfully improve their critical thinking skills. They interviewed more than 100 nurse leaders from academia, service settings, and professional associations and developed a list of core critical-thinking competencies in five broad categories: problem recognition, clinical decision-making, prioritization, clinical implementation, and reflection.

Characteristics of Critical Thinkers

Active listeners	Curious and insightful	Cognizant of rules of logic
Fair-minded	Humble	Realistic
Persistent	Honest with themselves and others	Team players
Good communicators		Creative
Open-minded	Proactive	Committed to excellence
Empathetic	Organized and systematic	*Source: Alfaro-LeFevre, 1999*
Independent thinkers	Flexible	

Precepting Critical Thinking

Alfaro-LeFevre (1999) has developed a list of critical-thinking key questions that can be used by a preceptor to help preceptees learn how to think critically:

- What major outcomes (observable results) do I/we hope to achieve?

- What problems or issues must be addressed to achieve the major outcomes?

- What are the circumstances (what is the context)?

- What knowledge is required?

- How much room is there for error?

- How much time do I/we have?

- What resources can help?

- Whose perspectives must be considered?

- What's influencing my thinking?

In addition, Alfaro-LeFevre (1999) offers suggestions on thinking critically about how to teach others:

- Be clear about the desired outcome.

- Decide what exactly the person must learn to achieve the desired outcome and decide the best way for the person to learn it.

- Reduce anxiety by offering support.

- Minimize distractions and teach at appropriate times.

- Use pictures, diagrams, and illustrations.

- Create mental images by using analogies and metaphors.

- Encourage people to remember by whatever words best trigger their mind.

- Keep it simple.

- Tune into your learners' responses; change the pace, techniques, or content if needed.

- Summarize key points.

Clinical Reasoning

Tanner (2006) defines *clinical reasoning* as "the processes by which nurses and other clinicians make their judgments, and includes both the deliberate process of generating alternatives, weighing them against the evidence, and choosing the most appropriate, and those patterns that might be characterized as engaged, practical reasoning (e.g., recognition of a pattern, an intuitive clinical grasp, a response without evident forethought)" (pp. 204-205).

Tanner (2006), in reviewing research on nurses and reasoning, found three interrelated patterns of reasoning that experienced nurses use in decision-making.

1. Analytic processes—Breaking a situation down into its elements; generating and systematically and rationally weighing alternatives against the data and potential outcomes.

2. Intuition—Immediately apprehending a situation (often using pattern recognition) as a result of experience with similar situations.

3. Narrative thinking—Thinking through telling and interpreting stories.

Facione and Facione (2008) discuss research in human reasoning that has found evidence of the function of two interconnected "systems" of reasoning. System 1 is "reactive, instinctive, quick, and holistic" and often "relies on highly expeditious heuristic maneuvers which can yield useful response to perceived problems without recourse to reflection" (Facione & Facione, 2008, p. 4). System 2, on the other hand, is described as "more deliberative, reflective, analytical, and procedural" and is "generally associated with reflective problem-solving and critical thinking" (p. 4). They note that the two systems never function completely independently and that, in some cases, the two systems actually offer somewhat of a corrective effect on each other. In fact, they say, "Effectively mixing System 1 and System 2 cognitive maneuvers to identify and resolve clinical problems is the normal form of mental processes involved in sound, expert critical thinking" (p. 5).

Simmons and colleagues (2003) investigated clinical reasoning of experienced (2-10 years) medical-surgical nurses. They found that the nurses used a number of thinking strategies (heuristics) that consolidated patient information and their knowledge and experience to speed their reasoning process. The most frequently used heuristics were:

- Recognizing a pattern or an inconsistency in the expected pattern
- Judging the value of the information about which they were reasoning
- Providing explanations for why they had reasoned as they had
- Forming relationships between data
- Drawing conclusions

Clinical Judgment

Critical thinking and clinical judgment are related. Facione and Facione (2008) describe the relationship as "critical thinking is the process we use to make a judgment about what to believe and what to do about the symptoms our patient is presenting for diagnosis and treatment" (p. 2).

Tanner (2006) defines *clinical judgment* to mean "an interpretation or conclusion about a patient's needs, concerns, or health problems, and/or the decision to take action (or not), use or modify standard approaches, or improvise new ones as deemed appropriate by the patient's response" (p. 204). Clinical judgment relies on knowing the patient in two ways— knowing the patient as a person and knowing the patient's pattern of responses (Tanner, Benner, Chesla, & Gordon, 1993).

Tanner (2006) has proposed a model of clinical judgment, based on a synthesis of the clinical judgment literature, that can be used in complex, rapidly changing patient situations. The model includes:

- Noticing—"A perceptual grasp of the situation at hand" (p. 208). Noticing, Tanner says, is "a function of nurses' expectations of the situation, whether they are explicit or not" and further that "these expectations stem from nurses' knowledge of the particular patient and his or her patterns of responses; their clinical or practical knowledge of similar patients, drawn from experience; and their textbook knowledge" (p. 208).

- Interpreting—"Developing a sufficient understanding of the situation to respond" (p. 208). Noticing triggers reasoning patterns that help nurses interpret the data and decide on a course of action.

- Responding—"Deciding on a course of action deemed appropriate for the situation, which may include 'no immediate action'" (p. 208).

- Reflecting—"Attending to the patients' responses to the nursing action while in the process of acting" (reflection in action) and "reviewing the outcomes of the action, focusing on the appropriateness of all of the preceding aspects (i.e., what was noticed, how it was interpreted, and how the nurse responded" (p. 208; reflection on action).

The use of this model can be helpful to preceptors as a structure for debriefing. It is a model of expert practice—what the new graduate aims for and what the experienced nurse needs to perfect. New graduate nurses have been shown to need major improvements in their clinical judgment skills. In reviewing 10 years of data using the Performance Based Development System (PBDS) for assessment, del Bueno (2005), found that only 35% of new graduates met the entry requirements (safe level) for clinical judgment, regardless of their pre-licensure educational preparation. They were unable to translate theory into practice. Accordingly, del Bueno posits that clinical practice with preceptors who ask questions (as opposed to giving answers) is the most critical intervention needed to improve the clinical judgment skills of new graduates.

Developing Expert Reasoning and Intuition

Malcolm Gladwell in his book *Blink* (2005) discusses the adaptive unconscious of the mind, which he describes as "a kind of giant computer that quickly and quietly processes a lot of the data we need in order to keep functioning as human beings" (p. 11) and a "decision-making apparatus that's capable of making very quick judgments based on very little information" (p. 12). The key themes of the research described in *Blink* are:

- Decisions made very quickly can be every bit as good as decisions made cautiously and deliberately.

- We have to learn when we should trust our instincts and when we should be wary of them.

- Our snap judgments and first impressions can be educated and controlled.

Gladwell describes what he calls "thin-slicing," "the ability of our unconscious to find patterns in situations and behavior based on very narrow slices of experience" (p. 23). In this case, the term "experience" is not being used, for example, to mean the long-term experience of caring for many patients of the same type, but rather "very narrow slices of experience" would refer to when you first walk into a patient's room and within seconds know that something does not fit the pattern you expect to see.

Gary Klein (1998) has studied nurses and other people who make decisions under time pressure when the stakes are high (i.e., firefighters, Navy SEALS, battlefield platoon leaders). Based on his research, he has found that what is generally termed "intuition" comes from experience, that we recognize things without knowing how we do the recognizing, and that what actually occurs is that we are drawn to certain cues because of situational awareness. He also notes, however, that because we often don't understand that we actually have experience behind "intuition," intuition gets discounted as hunches or guesses. His research, indeed, shows just the opposite. His findings indicate that the part of intuition that involves pattern matching and recognition of familiar and typical cases can be trained by expanding people's experience base.

Klein (1998) describes what he has termed the recognition-primed decision model, a model that brings together two processes, "the way decision makers size up the situation to recognize which course of action makes sense, and the way they evaluate the course of action by imagining it" (p. 24).

> Decision makers recognize the situation as typical and familiar . . . and proceed to take action. They understand what types of goals make sense (so priorities make sense), which cues are important (so there is not an overload of information), what to expect next (so they can prepare themselves and notice surprises, and the typical way of responding in a given situation. By recognizing a situation as typical, they also recognize a course of action likely to succeed. (p. 24)

This is compared to a rational choice strategy, which is similar to what we do in the nursing process. Though a rational choice strategy is often needed as a first step for novices or for initially working in teams to determine how everyone views the options, it is less useful with experts, who usually look for the first workable option in the current situation based on their knowledge and experience, and for high-risk situations that require rapid response.

Klein (1998) notes many things that experts can see that are invisible to others:

- Patterns that novices do not notice

- Anomalies, events that did not happen, and other violations of expectancies

- The big picture (situation awareness)

- The way things work

- Opportunities and improvisations

- Events that either already happened (the past) or are going to happen (the future)

- Differences that are too small for novices to notice

- Their own limitations (pp. 148-149)

In describing expert nursing, Dreyfus and Dreyfus (2009) note that experts use deliberative rationality—that is, when time permits, they think before they act, but normally, "they do not think about their rules for choosing goals or their reasons for choosing possible actions" (p. 16). Deliberative rationality (the kind of detached, meditative reflection exhibited by the expert when time permits thought), they say, "stands at the intersection of theory and practice. It is detached, reasoned observation of one's intuitive, practice-based behavior with an eye to challenging, and perhaps improving, intuition without replacing it by the purely theory-based action of the novice, advanced beginner, or competent performer" (pp. 17-18).

Confidence

Self-efficacy (confidence) is the belief of individuals in their capability to exercise some measure of control over their own functioning and over environmental events (Bandura, 1997). According to Bandura (2001), "Unless people believe they can produce desired results and forestall detrimental ones by their actions, they have little incentive to act or to persevere in the face of difficulties. Whatever other factors may operate as guides and motivators, they are rooted in the core belief that one has the power to produce effects by one's actions" (p. 10).

Rosabeth Moss Kanter (2006) notes that confidence consists of positive expectations for favorable outcomes and influences an individual's willingness to invest. "Confidence," she says, "is a sweet spot between arrogance and despair. Arrogance involves the failure to see any flaws or weaknesses, despair the failure to acknowledge any strengths" (p. 8).

Manojlovich (2005), in a study of predictors of professional nursing practice behaviors in hospital settings, found a significant relationship between self-efficacy to professional behaviors. Ulrich et al. (2010) found that self-confidence improved in new graduate nurses across and beyond an 18-week immersion RN residency that used one-to-one preceptors for new graduate nurses.

Helping preceptees develop confidence in themselves requires the use of many of the preceptor roles described in Chapter 1 and also requires the creation of a positive, enriching, and supportive learning environment. Competence and confidence are interrelated—each builds on, reinforces, and promotes the other.

Conclusion

Competence, critical thinking, clinical reasoning, clinical judgment, and confidence are all necessary components of any preceptorship. Role competence can be attained only by the connection of theory and practice. Critical thinking, clinical reasoning, and clinical judgment are the keys to making that happen. Competence without confidence is opportunity wasted. Preceptors are charged with helping preceptees master critical thinking, clinical reasoning, and clinical judgment skills so preceptees can move from novice to expert competency.

References

Alfaro-LeFevre, R. (1999). *Critical thinking in nursing: A practical approach* (2nd ed.). Philadelphia, PA: W.B. Saunders Company.

American Nurses Association (ANA). (2000). *Continuing competency: Nursing's agenda for the 21st century*. Washington, DC: Author.

American Nurses Association (ANA). (2003). *Nursing's social policy statement* (2nd ed.). Washington, DC: Author.

American Nurses Association (ANA). (2008). *Position statement: Professional role competence*. Washington, DC: Author.

American Nurses Association (ANA). (2010). *Nursing: Scope and standards of practice* (2nd ed.). Silver Spring, MD: Author.

American Philosophical Association. (1990). *Critical thinking: A statement of expert consensus for purposes of educational assessment and instruction*. ERIC Doc No. ED 315 423.

Bandura, A. (1997). *Self-efficacy: The exercise of control*. New York, NY: W.H. Freeman.

Bandura, A. (2001). Social cognitive theory: An agentic perspective. *Annual Review of Psychology, 52*, 1-26.

Berkow, S., Virkstis, K., Stewart, J., Aronson, S., & Donohue, M. (2011). Assessing individual frontline nurse critical thinking. *Journal of Nursing Administration, 41*(4), 168-171.

del Bueno, D.J. (2005). Why can't new registered nurse graduates think like nurses? *Nursing Education Perspectives, 26*(5), 278-282.

Dewey, J. (1933). *How we think: A restatement of the relation of reflective thinking to the education process*. Boston, MA: D.C. Heath.

Dreyfus, H. L., & Dreyfus, S. E. (2009). The relationship of theory and practice in the acquisition of skill. In P. Benner, C. Tanner, & C. Chelsa (Eds.), *Expertise in nursing practice: Caring, clinical judgment, and ethics* (2nd ed., pp. 1-24). New York, NY: Springer Publishing Company.

Facione, N. C., & Facione, P. A. (1996). Externalizing the critical thinking in knowledge development and clinical judgment. *Nursing Outlook, 44*(3), 129-136.

Facione, N. C., & Facione, P. A. (2008). Critical thinking and clinical judgment. In N. C. Facione & P. A. Facione (Eds.), *Critical thinking and clinical reasoning in the health sciences: A teaching anthology* (pp. 1-13). Millbrae, CA: The California Academic Press.

Facione, P. A. (1990). *Critical thinking: A statement of expert consensus for purposes of educational assessment and instruction*. Millbrae, CA: The California Academic Press. Retrieved from http://www.insightassessment.com/CT-Resources/Expert-Consensus-on-Critical-Thinking

Facione, P. A. (2011). *Critical thinking: What it is and why it counts*. Millbrae, CA: The California Academic

Press. Retrieved from http://www.insightassessment.com/CT-Resources

Gladwell, M. (2005). *Blink: The power of thinking without thinking*. New York, NY: Little, Brown and Company.

Jackson, M. (2006). Defining the concept of critical thinking. In M. Jackson, D. D. Ignatavicius, & B. Case (Eds.), *Conversations in critical thinking and clinical judgment* (pp. 3-18), Sudbury, MA: Jones and Bartlett Publishers.

Kanter, R. M. (2006). *Confidence: How winning streaks & losing streaks begin & end*. New York, NY: Three Rivers Press.

Kearney, M. H., & Kenward, K. (2010). Nurses' competence development during the first 5 years of practice. *Journal of Nursing Regulation*, *1*(1), 9-15.

Klein, G. (1998). *Sources of power: How people make decisions*. Boston, MA: Massachusetts Institute of Technology.

Lenburg, C. (1999). The frameworks, concepts and methods of the competency outcomes and performances assessment (COPA). *The Online Journal of Issues in Nursing*, *4*(2), Manuscript 2.

Manojlovich, M. (2005). Predictors of professional nursing practice behaviors in hospital settings. *Nursing Research*, *54*(1), 41-47.

Paul, R. W., & Heaslip, P. (1995). Critical thinking and intuitive nursing practice. *Journal of Advanced Nursing*, *22*(1), 40-47.

Scheffer, B. K., & Rubenfeld, M. G. (2000). A consensus statement on critical thinking in nursing. *Journal of Nursing Education*, *39*(8), 352-359.

Simmons, B., Lanuza, D., Fonteyn, M., Hicks, F., & Holm, K. (2003). Clinical reasoning in experienced nurses. *Western Journal of Nursing Research*, *25*(6), 701-719.

Tanner, C. A. (2006). Thinking like a nurse: A research-based model of clinical judgment in nursing. *Journal of Nursing Education*, *45*(6), 204-211.

Tanner, C. A., Benner, P., Chesla, C., & Gordon, D. R. (1993). The phenomenology of knowing the patient. *Journal of Nursing Scholarship*, *25*(4), 273-280.

Ulrich, B., Krozek, C., Early, S., Ashlock, C. H., Africa, L. M., & Carman, M. L. (2010). Improving retention, confidence, and competence of new graduate nurses: Results from a 10-year longitudinal database. *Nursing Economic$*, *28*(6), 363-376.

Preceptor Development Plan: Competence, Critical Thinking, Clinical Reasoning, Clinical Judgment, and Confidence

Review the information on competence, critical thinking, clinical reasoning, clinical judgment, and confidence described in this chapter. What are your strengths? In which areas do you need to increase your knowledge and expertise? What is your plan for expanding your knowledge and expertise? What resources are available? Who can help you?

Review the competencies that are required for your preceptee. If written descriptions of these competencies are not available, work with other stakeholders to develop them. Assess your own knowledge and expertise on each of the competencies. What are your strengths? In which areas do you need to increase your knowledge and expertise? What is your plan for expanding your knowledge and expertise? What resources are available? Who can help you?

Name:			
Competence Assessment			
Strengths	Needs	Plan	Resources
Competence Development			
Strengths	Needs	Plan	Resources
Critical Thinking			
Strengths	Needs	Plan	Resources
Clinical Reasoning			
Strengths	Needs	Plan	Resources

Clinical Judgment			
Strengths	Needs	Plan	Resources
Confidence			
Strengths	Needs	Plan	Resources

Note: This form and other resources are available at www.RNPreceptor.com.

Preceptor Development Plan Preceptee Role Competencies				
Role:				
Competency	**Preceptee Strengths**	**Preceptee Needs**	**Plan**	**Resources**

Note: This form and other resources are available at www.RNPreceptor.com.

"If you're not sure where you're going, you're liable to end up someplace else."

–Robert Mager

Having a Plan: Developing and Using Objectives, Goals, and Outcomes

5

Karen C. Robbins, MS, RN, CNN

Mary S. Haras, MS, MBA, APN, NP-C, CNN

OBJECTIVES

- Distinguish the differences among goals, objectives, and outcomes

- Discuss different learning taxonomies and their application to the preceptorship process

- Create related goals, objectives, and outcomes

A nurse entering a new position, either as a new graduate nurse or a nurse with experience moving into another practice area, will need to become familiar with and competent in the new practice area and/or role. Preceptors are the key in assuring that this occurs. Goals, objectives, and outcomes form the road map for the work of the preceptor and the preceptee. They can be written and/or verbal and should be agreed upon by the preceptor and preceptee. As a preceptor, you need to know the goals of the institution, as well as those of the preceptee. Buy-in and acceptance will facilitate the best preceptor-preceptee relationship.

This chapter focuses on the development of measurable goals, objectives, and outcomes; how the preceptor and preceptee can interact to achieve them; and the tools with which these accomplishments can be measured. The preceptor and preceptee both need to understand these principles so that the precepting experience is focused and can be measured. Said another way, you will not know when you have achieved the aim of the precepting experience if the target is not defined.

Expectations

The transfer of learning and application into practice is ultimately the goal of a precepting experience (Su, Osisek, & Starnes, 2004). Preceptors are expected to provide the needed experiences with accompanying oversight so the preceptee can become competent. In keeping with adult learning principles, learning should progress from simple to complex (Nesbitt, 2006). Three questions must be answered to meet these needs:

- What does the preceptee need to learn?

- What approaches will be used to promote learning?

- How will success be measured and identified? (Su et al., 2004)

Glennon (2006) distinguishes outcomes from objectives in the following statement: "Outcomes relate directly to professional practice; objectives relate to instruction" (p. 55). The American Association of Colleges of Nursing (AACN, 2008) baccalaureate essentials document defines outcome as a "broad performance indicator, related to the knowledge, skills, and attitudes, needed by a baccalaureate graduate" (p. 38). From the time that an individual enters a nursing program, the process of preceptorship begins, with the ultimate goal of providing the graduate nurse the ability to care for complex, diverse, and changing patient populations and/or developing skills in specialties such as education and management. The National Nursing Staff Development Organization (NNSDO) states that the development of desired outcomes should involve the learners and the key stakeholders (ANA & NNSDO, 2010). Hence, learner objectives and outcomes should be discussed between the preceptor and preceptee from the outset and throughout the preceptorship experience, so that expectations are clear and are consistent with the overall goals of the program.

In an ideal world, all preceptorships would have preplanned objectives and outcomes, but this is not always the case. In addition, precepting occurs in the dynamic setting of a hospital, where precepting plans often go awry because of the needs of the patients. At times you have to abandon the objectives agreed upon for a given time frame because of the circumstances of the day, the assignment, or responsibilities. Preceptors sometimes need to adjust the intended activities "on the fly" as situations arise. For example, a preceptor might be planning to work with a manager preceptee on the process of performance reviews when a clinical emergency arises and demands the involvement of the preceptor and preceptee. This provides valuable experience for the manager's role in the situation even though it deviates from the agreed-upon activity. To have this flexibility, preceptors must understand the concepts behind the development, use, and evaluation of goals, objectives, and outcomes.

The Relationship Among Goals, Objectives, and Outcomes

Goals serve as the overreaching purpose of the activity—the aim, or the endpoint. The goal is the final, global outcome of the teaching-learning process (Bastable & Doody, 2008). Goals are what drive the actions of the nurse, the unit/department, and the hospital/ organization. Goals are forward-thinking and must be clearly stated so that the objectives and outcomes that follow can be articulated in such a way as to achieve the ultimate goal. The interrelationship among goals, objectives, and outcomes is shown in Figure 5.1. The term *goal* is sometimes used synonymously, although incorrectly, with the term *objective*. Goals are accomplished over weeks or months and incorporate a number of specific objectives and outcomes that are met during that time (Bastable & Doody, 2008). For the preceptee, the goal might be to become a competent nurse or a competent educator. For the preceptor, the goal might be to serve as a role model for newer nurses. For the unit/department, the goal of the preceptorship program might be to improve staff morale and decrease turnover. For the institution, the goal might be improved quality of patient care. Regardless of the goal, it must be clearly stated, be important to the involved parties, and be realistic.

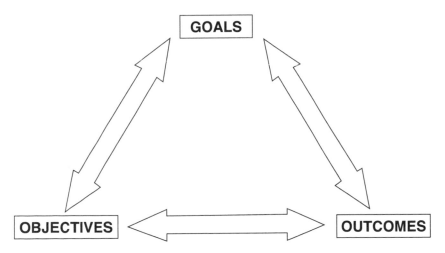

Figure 5.1   Interrelationship Among Goals, Outcomes, and Objectives.

Objectives vs. Outcomes

Objectives have guided education since the 1950s, when Benjamin Bloom released his taxonomy of educational objectives (Glennon, 2006). Objectives are teaching- and content-focused, short-term, and action-oriented. Outcomes are learning- and student-focused, more long-term, and behaviorally oriented. Both are important in a preceptor-preceptee relationship, and you cannot have one without the other. Outcome statements require the blending of several domains of knowledge to achieve a higher level of functioning, as is necessary in the complexity of nursing care today (Glennon, 2006). As the paradigm shifts in the context of fiscal concerns in the clinical arena, outcomes might be assessed in monetary terms, as well as in patient safety, health achievement, or the productivity of education initiatives. The question might become whether the resources required support the outcomes (Wittman-Price & Fasolka, 2010). Objectives and outcomes survive the test of time, however, as they are parsimonious and encapsulate the complexity of the teaching/learning process (Wittman-Price & Fasolka, 2010).

Objectives and outcomes both use behavioral terms, but outcomes are broader and reflect the evolution from learning to performing. Outcome format/verbiage states that "at the end of the session, the preceptee will be able to . . . " as opposed to simply stating that "the preceptee will . . . " (Wittman-Price & Fasolka, 2010), thereby establishing a direct link between the "session" and the outcome. The learner, the behavior, and the content are common elements of both. Ultimately, knowledge and skills development must support the ability for nurses to practice safely, and there must be a formal means to measure or observe the nurses' achievement of their stated outcomes. Goals and objectives remain the common verbiage in the various taxonomies when discussing the interaction between a preceptor and preceptee. Specificity is needed in this process to clearly articulate the expectations of the experience. Weekly goals provide a vehicle to monitor progress toward increased complexity in work and in areas needing additional attention and to reinforce what has been learned (Duclos-Miller, 2006).

Buy-in from the outset is a critical element for a successful preceptorship. The preceptor and preceptee must agree upon the goals and how to accomplish the objectives and must keep track of the progress of putting the pieces together and completing the puzzle. Toward that end, the goals and objectives must be realistic, as failure to establish realistic goals will set all parties up for failure. These goals and objectives are focused upon what the preceptee is expected to be able to do, not upon what the preceptor is expected to teach. The objectives provide the map to reach the destination: the goal. Applying the primary learning taxonomies to the preceptor-preceptee learning process is an integral part of this.

Learning Taxonomies

Simply stated, a *taxonomy* is a classification for information or a mechanism that categorizes how things relate to each other (Bastable & Doody, 2008; Forehand, 2005). "Learners have different preferred ways of taking in information, such as verbally or visually, and for processing that information, like manipulating something or thinking about details before acting" (Ullrich & Hafer, 2009, p. 89). Because adult learners do not all learn the same way, it is sometimes necessary to alter the teaching approach to be effective. Preceptors have a number of learning taxonomies available to guide development of the teaching-learning interaction. Each approaches the process differently.

Bloom's Taxonomy: Objectives and Domains of Learning

Bloom's (1956) taxonomy classifies cognitive learning objectives and is perhaps one of the most widely cited tools and references in education (Forehand, 2005). Bloom's three domains of learning are cognitive, affective, and psychomotor (Bastable & Doody, 2008; Bloom, 1956; Forehand, 2005; Waller, 2001). Each of the domains in this taxonomy has multiple levels and is illustrated in Figure 5.2 (Churches, 2009). The first of these, the *cognitive domain*, is known as the thinking domain and is further divided into six hierarchical levels: knowledge, comprehension, application, analysis, synthesis, and evaluation (Bastable & Doody, 2008; Forehand, 2005; Waller, 2001). This is predicated on the fact that the hierarchy is described as a stairway. It encourages the preceptee to climb to the higher or the next level of thought, so that someone functioning at the analytical level has mastered those levels preceding it, i.e., knowledge, comprehension, and application (Forehand, 2005).

The *affective domain* addresses attitudes, feelings, beliefs, and emotions (Neumann & Forsyth, 2008) and is sometimes referred to as the feeling domain (Bastable & Doody, 2008). This is a more difficult domain for the preceptor, because it does not rely upon facts or principles (the cognitive domain) or motor skills (the psychomotor domain) that are measured more easily (Neumann & Forsyth, 2008). Learning in this domain is a long-term process and might be more difficult to learn for nurses who are less aware of their own value system (Neumann & Forsyth, 2008). This might, however, present an opportunity for preceptees to become more aware of their own values and attitudes (Bastable & Doody, 2008). Preceptors play a key role in helping preceptees identify their values and attitudes by asking probing questions and using role-play, case studies, and critical reflection.

The affective domain consists of five levels and considers the depth of a person's emotional responses to tasks, in contrast to the cognitive domain, which looks at complexity of behaviors (Bastable & Doody, 2008). Objectives are more difficult to write in the affective domain because these behaviors tend to be less tangible and, therefore, not as easily measured. The personal value system of an individual, however, must be consistent with the values of the profession. The American Nurses Association (ANA) Code of Ethics for Nurses with Interpretive Statements is an example of a source for professional values (ANA, 2001). These tenets affirm the ethical obligations and duties for anyone entering the nursing profession, reflect the understanding of nursing's commitment to society, and are nonnegotiable (ANA, 2001). The mission, vision, and model of care reflect the culture and values of an organization and also fall in the affective domain of learning (Neumann & Forsyth, 2008).

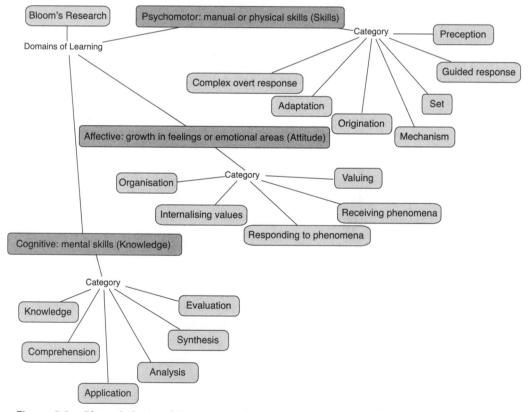

Figure 5.2   Bloom's Original Taxonomy identifies the domains of learning and represents a hierarchy. It begins with the cognitive domain (lower left), and progresses through the affective and psychomotor domains. Not only are the domains in a hierarchy, but there is also a progression of skills within each domain, as shown here.

Used with permission. Churches, 2009

Skills are addressed in the six levels of the *psychomotor domain* (Bastable & Doody, 2008; Churches, 2009; Forehand, 2005; Waller, 2001). Fine and gross motor abilities requiring increasingly complex actions fall under this domain. The goals and objectives in this domain focus more upon the skill itself, rather than acquiring new knowledge. A preceptor, for example, should not ask questions from the cognitive domain when working with a psychomotor skill, because that might shift the preceptee's focus away from the skill. Instead, the preceptee should have the opportunity to practice the skill and then demonstrate successful mastery of that skill. This is the "hands on" component of the preceptor-preceptee relationship and is critical to the integration of knowledge and skill for the preceptee. As preceptees gain the knowledge, skills, and attributes to become proficient, they move along the continuum from objective to outcome to goal achievement.

The Revised Bloom's Taxonomy (RBT; also referred to as the Anderson et al. Cognitive Revised Domain, or the Anderson/Bloom Taxonomy; O'Neil & Murphy, 2010) was released in 2001. The greatest changes can be seen in the areas of terminology, structure, and emphasis (Forehand, 2005; see Figures 5.3 and 5.4). The biggest change is in the wording, changing nouns to action verbs, and it is applicable for a much broader audience (Forehand, 2005). The original lowest level, knowledge, was changed to remembering, based upon the notion that if you cannot remember something, you cannot apply knowledge or concepts to understand it (Churches, 2008, 2009). The two highest levels were changed from synthesis and evaluation to evaluating and creating. You must be able to evaluate (that is, judge or test) something before being able to devise or invent (that is, to create). You must be able to analyze and evaluate the efficacy for specific nursing interventions before being able to devise a new plan of care. Note that these two functions (evaluate and devise) are hierarchal and are dependent upon one's ability to complete the lower levels before progressing to these higher-level functions. Churches (2009), however, states that the learning can begin at any point when the lower levels of the taxonomy are included in a scaffolded learning task. Scaffolding is a metaphor for the preceptor's guidance to support the preceptee as the preceptee progresses in skills accomplishment. As the preceptee advances, the preceptor slowly withdraws direction and support, enabling the preceptee to become independent in the newly acquired skill or knowledge (Lipscom, Swanson, & West, 2004). Scaffolding can enhance the progression of lower order thinking skills (LOTS) to higher order thinking skills (HOTS; Churches, 2009). The changes in the hierarchy of LOTS to HOTS, not only in verbiage but in reversing the order of the top two levels in the revised iteration, are shown in Figures 5.3 and 5.4.

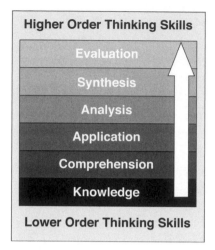

Flgure 5.3   Bloom's Original Taxonomy illustrates the progression in the taxonomy of lower order thinking skills to higher order thinking skills, as compared to the Revised Bloom's Taxonomy.

Used with permission. Churches, 2009

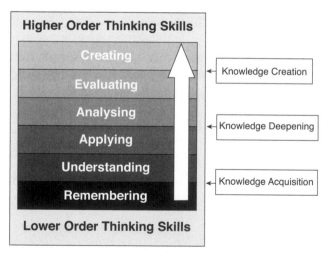

Figure 5.4   The Revised Bloom's Taxonomy reflects the change in verbiage from nouns to verbs and a change in the order of lower order thinking skills to higher order thinking skills. The progression of knowledge depicted on the right represents the ascension of higher order thinking skills necessary to advance beyond remembering and understanding, that is, the ability to critically think.

Used with permission. Churches, 2009

The Revised Bloom's Taxonomy adds a second dimension of knowledge to each of the three domains, where the unidimensional original taxonomy considered only the domains of learning and did not consider the factual, conceptual, procedural, and metacognitive forms of knowledge. These two dimensions of the knowledge to be learned by the preceptees and the cognitive processes to help preceptors in their interactions, along with sample verbs in each category, are shown in Table 5.1. Examples of the verbs in ascension of the affective domain are found in Table 5.2.

Table 5.1   Revised Bloom's Taxonomy: Knowledge and Cognitive Processes

Knowledge Dimension	Cognitive Process Dimension					
	Remember	Understand	Apply	Analyze	Evaluate	Create
Factual	Define, list, recall	Calculate, identify, report	Classify, solve, use	Test, compare, infer	Judge, appraise, verify	Change, design, predict
Conceptual	Describe	Interpret	Experiment	Explain	Assess	Plan
Procedural	Tabulate	Predict	Calculate	Differentiate	Conclude	Compose
Metacognitive	Appropriate use	Execute	Construct	Achieve	Action	Actualize

Sources: Forehand, 2005; O'Neill & Murphy, 2010; Oregon State University, 2011

Table 5.2   Revised Bloom's Taxonomy: Affective Domain

Level	Examples of Verbs
Receiving	Ask, reply, accept
Valuing	Justify, propose, relinquish
Organization and Conceptualization	Arrange, balance, theorize
Characterization by Value	Discriminate, question, change

Source: O'Neill & Murphy, 2010

Bloom did not fully develop the psychomotor domain when the taxonomy was released in 1956, and others have adapted and expanded upon it (Davis, Chen, & Cambell, 2010; O'Neill & Murphy, 2010). One example is the work of Elizabeth Simpson, who adapted and further developed this domain in 1972 (Bastable & Doody, 2008; O'Neill & Murphy, 2010; Simpson, 1972).

Four orderly steps are common to the various iterations of the psychomotor domain: observing, imitating, practicing, and adapting (Bastable & Doody, 2008). Simpson's taxonomy contains seven progressive steps. The first step is *perception*. As the name implies, a sensory awareness prompts the preceptee about a task to be performed. This could include observing a procedure being performed or perhaps reading the steps in a procedure. *Set* indicates the ability of the preceptee to follow directions and a readiness to learn. Imitation of a skill with coaching or direction from the preceptor is *guided response*, that is, the preceptee would be performing the task with the preceptor's oversight. If inserting an intravenous (IV) line is the task at hand for the preceptee, *mechanism* would indicate that some type of preparation had been performed, for example, viewing a recording of the steps and/or reviewing them with the preceptor, or performing this with the preceptor. With this step, the preceptee begins to demonstrate some ability to perform the skill with little conscious effort. When the preceptee is able to perform the IV insertion confidently, efficiently, and seemingly automatically, this is the *complex overt response*, the fifth of the seven levels. When less than ideal circumstances are present, the preceptee achieves the level of *adaptation* when the IV is inserted despite obstacles to which the preceptee must adapt, for example, determining how to place the IV in a patient with limited sites. *Origination*, the highest level of the psychomotor domain, might be the development of a skill by placing an IV with the nondominant hand because of possible barriers, for example, a hand injury to the dominant hand.

A list of sample verbs that are present in the psychomotor domain is shown in Table 5.3. Remember that the preceding levels are prerequisite behaviors to progress through the hierarchy.

Andrew Churches (2009) has identified action verbs for the Revised Bloom's Taxonomy, as shown in Table 5.4, with a progression of low order thinking skills (LOTS) to high order thinking skills (HOTS). The higher levels are needed for the creation of new knowledge, not merely remembering information, as happens at the LOTS level.

Churches considered these verbs in the context of classroom activities and suggests these do not adequately reflect the emergence of multiple forms of communication technology. Accordingly, he has proposed Bloom's Digital Taxonomy (see Figure 5.5). The column on the right of the image titled "Communication Spectrum" is indicative of the significant role that communication has in learning. Collaborating is one of the skills under the Communication Spectrum, and Churches has proposed that not only is it a 21st century skill, it is essential for collaboration in this century. An expanded discussion of the digital taxonomy can be found on Churches' website (Churches, 2009).

Table 5.3   Psychomotor Domain: Examples of Verbs

Level	Examples of Verbs
Perception	Chooses, describes, differentiates, identifies, relates, recognizes, selects, separates
Set	Arranges, begins, displays, prepares, reacts, recognize, responds, shows, starts
Guided response	Assembles, builds, calibrates, dismantles, follows, lifts, manipulates, measures, mixes, pours, responds, simulates, transfers
Mechanism	Assembles, constructs, grasps, manipulates, measures, mixes, organizes, performs
Complex overt response	Assembles, builds, calibrates, coordinates, demonstrates, makes, mixes, organizes
Adaptation	Adapts, adjusts, alters, conforms, converts, integrates, rearranges, reconciles, regulates, revises, standardizes, substitutes
Origination	Arranges, combines, creates, designs, reformulates, trouble-shoots

Sources: Simpson, 1966-67; University of Mississippi, n.d.

Table 5.4   Lower Order Thinking Skills (LOTS) to Higher Order Thinking Skills (HOTS)—Sample Verbs

Lower Order Thinking Skills (LOTS)

Remembering—Recognizing, listing, describing, identifying, retrieving, naming, locating, finding

Understanding—Interpreting, summarizing, inferring, paraphrasing, classifying, comparing, explaining, exemplifying

Applying—Implementing, carrying out, using, executing

Analyzing—Comparing, organizing, deconstructing, attributing, outlining, finding, structuring, integrating

Evaluating—Checking, hypothesizing, critiquing, experimenting, judging, testing, detecting, monitoring

Creating—Designing, constructing, planning, producing, inventing, devising, making

Higher Order Thinking Skills (HOTS)

Used with permission. Churches, 2009

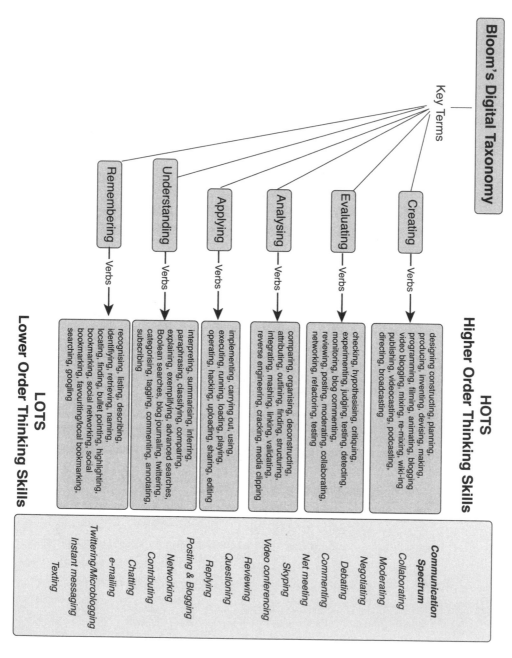

Figure 5.5   Bloom's Digital Taxonomy

Used with permission. Churches, 2009

Fink's Taxonomy of Significant Learning

Most nurses and nurse educators are comfortable and familiar with the taxonomies of Bloom and Anderson, but might be unfamiliar with Fink's (2003) taxonomy of significant learning. Fink's taxonomy emerged from his recognition of important kinds of learning beyond the cognitive domain, based on his definition of learning as a change in the learner. It is well recognized that one of the major roles of the preceptor is to help socialize new nurses to their roles in the organization (Baltimore, 2004; Burns & Northcutt, 2009; Murphy, 2008; Smedley, Morey, & Race, 2010), which is congruent with Fink's belief that "significant learning requires that there be some kind of lasting change that is important in terms of the learner's life" (Fink, 2003, p. 30).

Fink describes six major categories of significant learning (foundational knowledge, application, integration, human dimension, caring, and learning how to learn) that are meaningful to the learner and provide a framework for the preceptor-preceptee relationship (see Figure 5.6).

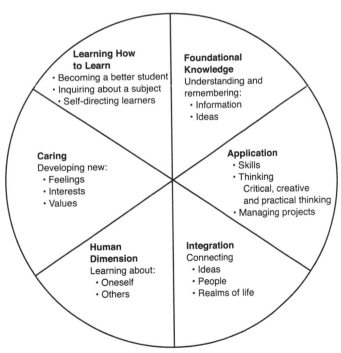

Figure 5.6   Fink's Taxonomy of Learning Styles

Used with permission. Fink, 2003

This taxonomy is not hierarchical, but is relational and interactive. When one type of learning occurs, it becomes easier for the learner to see the significance of other components of the learning process and their application to themselves or others (see Figure 5.7).

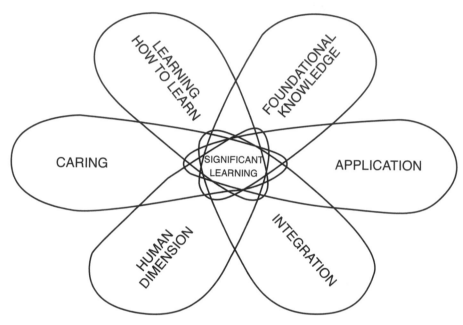

Figure 5.7   Fink's Taxonomy of Significant Learning
Used with permission. Fink, 2003

Fink's category of *foundational knowledge* assures that preceptees have a basic understanding of the relevant ideas and information in their new area of practice. Through formal learning activities, repetition, and performance review, preceptees will strengthen their understanding and remembrance of the specific information necessary to safely practice.

Application includes socialization to the unit and organization, as well as prioritization of patient assignments; critical, creative, and practical thinking; and skill utilization. It "allows other kinds of learning to become useful" (Fink, 2003, p. 31). Besides fostering socialization, preceptors encourage their preceptees to be self-directed to develop necessary critical thinking skills (Murphy, 2008). The value of application learning is in the development of communication skills and learning how to manage complex patient situations. Some examples of questions that the preceptor can ask of the preceptee to stimulate the three kinds of thinking—critical thinking, creative thinking, and practical thinking—are shown in Table 5.5.

Table 5.5 Sample Preceptor Questions to Stimulate Three Types of Thinking for Preceptee		
Critical Thinking	*Creative Thinking*	*Practical Thinking*
Compare and contrast Type 1 and Type 2 diabetes.	Draw the pathophysiology of diabetes and its complications.	What lesson does diabetes provide for patients today?
In what ways are patients on hemodialysis and peritoneal dialysis similar?	How might you encourage a patient to accept dialysis?	Why do patients choose a particular treatment modality?

Integration learning enables the preceptee to make the necessary connections between things. This might be between ideas, concepts, procedures, people, or realms of life (work and home, work and school, etc.). By making new connections, the nurse gains intellectual power and self-confidence. One major kind of connection is that of connecting academic work with other areas of life. This involves the preceptor helping the preceptee build the connection with the theory learned in class or school and real-life patient situations.

Learning in the *human dimension* enables nurses to learn new things about themselves and others. The nurse develops emotional intelligence as described by Daniel Goleman (1998). Goleman has described personal competence to include self-awareness, self-regulation, and motivation, and social competence as empathy and social skills. The preceptor is key in this process by asking important questions to the preceptee; providing relevant, meaningful feedback about the preceptee's performance; and serving as a role model. The preceptee is then better able to understand why and how a patient/family acts and how to more effectively interact with others.

Caring as a result of a learning experience increases the depth or manner in which the preceptee cares about something. Preceptees now have the energy to learn more and integrate it into their daily life. They might have new feelings or values as a result of their learned experience. Preceptors can facilitate this process by asking preceptees, "What is the most important thing you would like to get out of this experience?" The preceptor can be asked, "What do you want your preceptee to get excited about?" By paying attention to responses and looking for key words such as *enjoy, like, amazed by,* and *fascinated by,* the preceptor can see that the preceptee has developed feelings for a subject and that values have emerged that might not have been there before.

Finally, through the course of the preceptorship experience, the preceptee is *learning how to learn.* The preceptee learns how to be a better student and learns how to add knowledge specific to nursing. This commits the preceptee to lifelong learning and the ability to learn more effectively. The preceptee might learn how to report using handoff procedures or learn ways to become more self-directed in identifying learning needs.

Because Fink's taxonomy is relational and interactive, the preceptor also works through the six categories of learning. Both the preceptee and preceptor learn from each other, and significant learning occurs. Fink's taxonomy has two major implications for preceptors: First, the learning goals must incorporate yet exceed content mastery and, second, the preceptor must use a combination of goals to create interaction effects to enhance significant learning by the preceptee (Fink, 2003).

Behavioral Objectives

Bastable and Doody (2008) have described the pros and cons of using behavioral objectives. Though behavioral objectives are not a magic potion, they do provide a vehicle to address the issues of planning, implementing, and evaluating the teaching-learning experience. Some of the advantages and disadvantages of behavioral objectives are described in Table 5.6. When reviewing the pros and cons, it seems clear that behavioral objectives might not be applicable in all situations. Their advantages, however, underscore their benefits more than their disadvantages detract from them.

Table 5.6   Advantages and Disadvantages of Behavioral Objectives
Advantages
They help to keep the preceptor and preceptee focused.
Colleagues will know what is planned for the learning experience.
They clarify the expectations for the preceptee.
They enhance organization of the teaching material to stay on track.
They foster analysis of the content so that the preceptor scrutinizes the material being covered.
They individualize the approaches for the preceptee's unique needs.
They focus upon the outcome of the teaching-learning experience, not the process.
They identify behaviors to be accomplished that will demonstrate success (or failure) to achieve the particular objective.
Disadvantages
They might be superfluous for a person whose expertise at assessing the preceptee's needs does not require their use.

Table 5.6   Advantages and Disadvantages of Behavioral Objectives (cont.)

Disadvantages

The "big picture" might be lost when the activity is diminished into smaller parts.

The time required to construct them does not justify the benefit in writing them.

They are an exercise in pedagogy, focusing upon the preceptor's expectations rather than the preceptee's ability to be self-directed.

Their use can suffocate creativity, forcing the preceptor to focus upon specific activities.

Nursing is multifaceted, and their use cannot comprehensively address all aspects of care.

Complex cognitive skills cannot be easily observed or measured and, hence, not adequately captured by behavioral objectives.

Source: Bastable & Doody, 2008

Creating Outcome Statements

Competency outcome statements can guide the clinical experience and establish a foundation upon which the actions of the preceptee can be assessed (Glennon, 2006). According to Bresciani (n.d.), "It is important to define and clearly express the mission and objectives of the program or process that you want to assess" (p. 1). Bresciani identified six questions that must be answered. We provide the answers.

Q: *Why is the assessment being conducted?*

A: To measure the clinical competence of the preceptee in achieving the outcomes of the teaching-learning process.

Q: *For whom is the assessment being done?*

A: The preceptee. Note: Again, this is focused upon the behaviors of the preceptee, not the actions of the preceptor.

Q: *How will the results be used?*

A: To monitor the measurable progress of the preceptee through the teaching-learning process. To determine when/if the preceptee is competent to perform safely and effectively for the specific role.

Q: *To whom and in what format will the results be shared?*

A: A clinical competency tool and/or weekly goals, for example, will document the progression throughout the teaching-learning experience. The achievement of objectives first and then measurement of the outcomes will determine when the goals have been achieved. This will be shared with the manager or appropriate supervisory person to document these accomplishments.

Q: *When and how often will the assessments be conducted?*

A: This will depend upon the policies and practice of the individual organization and the needs of the preceptee.

Q: *What decisions will be made based upon the findings?*

A: The status of the achievement of outcomes and goals will determine whether the preceptor-preceptee relationship can be terminated or if it needs to continue beyond the predetermined time frame.

Distinguishing Outcomes From Objectives

A practice-centered learning experience enhances the preceptee's ownership of the teaching-learning experience (Glennon, 2006). Distinctions between outcomes and objectives are shown in Table 5.7.

Table 5.7	Distinctions Between Outcomes and Objectives	
Dimension	**Outcomes**	**Objectives**
Conceptual	Whole	Situation at a point in time
Descriptors	Complex	Tasks
	Interrelationships	Skill
	Unite several themes	Discrete points of knowing
Orientation	Results-focused	Process-focused
	Student-oriented	Teacher-oriented
	Learning-focused	Content-focused
	Related to professional	Related to academic achievement practice

Adapted from Glennon, 2006

Developing Measurable Objectives and Outcomes

Preceptees need well-developed behavioral objectives that are clear and concise and articulate, measurable outcomes that are demonstrated as a result of the teaching-learning experience (Bastable & Doody, 2008). Mager (1997) identifies three characteristics that are important to accomplish this.

1. **Performance**—Visible actions the preceptee is expected to perform that demonstrate the accomplishment of the objectives. "The preceptee inserts an IV without assistance."

2. **Condition**—Depicts the situation, resources, or constraints under which the preceptee will demonstrate the behavior. "The preceptee gathers appropriate equipment needed to take to the patient to start an IV."

3. **Criterion**—Expresses the time frame, accuracy, or how well the behavior will be demonstrated to assure sufficient mastery of the competency being measured, that is, the level of competence that is expected. "The preceptee will successfully initiate an IV in four of five patients by the end of the third week of orientation."

Waller (2001) has identified four common elements that the actual structure of an objective contains: action verb, conditions, standard, and intended audience, in this case, the preceptee. The most important component is the action verb; one must always use an action verb because it declares what the preceptee will be able to do as a result of the learning experience. An easy way of remembering these four elements of a behavioral objective is the "ABCD rule," audience, behavior, condition, and degree (Bastable & Doody, 2008; Heinich, Molenda, Russell, & Smaldino, 2001).

ABCD Rule for Developing Objectives

A—Audience (for whom is the statement written)

B—Behavior (what is the expected action)

C—Condition (what are the circumstances in which this is to occur)

D—Degree (how much and to what extent)

Sources: Bastable & Doody, 2008; Heinrich et al., 2001

Another model that is useful for both objectives and outcomes is the *SMART* rule, because it lends itself to a variety of audiences and settings. Several interpretations of the acronym exist, as shown in the following list (Bastable & Doody, 2008; University of Central Florida & Seminole Community College, 2008).

> **Specific**—Specifies what is to be accomplished in clear and definite terms; describes abilities, knowledge, values, attitudes, and performance; use of strong action verbs.
>
> **Measurable**—Can be assessed in more than one way; quantify or qualify objectives, for example, percentage amounts, cost, numeric.
>
> **Achievable, Attainable**—Is it realistic? The outcome might move the system forward.
>
> **Realistic, Results-Oriented**—Describe the standards that are expected; can the objectives be achieved with available resources?
>
> **Timely, Time-bound**—Specify the time period in which this is to be achieved.

The following example demonstrates the application of these very similar concepts in an objective stated earlier: "The preceptee (intended audience or audience) will successfully initiate an IV (action verb, behavior, specific) in four of five patients (standard, degree, or measurable) by the end of the third week of orientation (condition, timely)."

The acronym of *MATURE* (University of Central Florida & Seminole Community College, 2008) has also been used to describe the process of assessing student learning outcomes. This could easily be adapted to successfully assess learning objectives.

> **Matches**—Directly related to the outcome it is measuring
>
> **Appropriate methods**—Uses appropriate direct and indirect measures
>
> **Targets**—Indicates desired level of performance
>
> **Useful**—Measures help identify what to improve
>
> **Reliable**—Based on tested, known methods
>
> **Effective and Efficient**—Concisely characterizes the outcome

Pitfalls of Developing Objectives

Saying that objectives should be clear and concise means that they should be open to few interpretations. When the action is a clear performance verb (for example, classify, demonstrate, explain, or recall), you leave little room for misinterpretation. The prescribed action is apparent. Verbs that reflect more abstract actions (for example, understand or appreciate) are not as easily observed but inferred from related actions. Verbs that connote thinking, feeling, and believing should be avoided because of the difficulty observing them (Bastable & Doody, 2008). The lists in Table 5.8 are examples of verbs that have few interpretations, desirable in that they leave little room for interpretation, and verbs that are vague, not easily measurable and, therefore, not desirable.

Table 5.8 Examples of Verbs With Few or Too Many Interpretations	
Verbs With Few Interpretations (Advised)	*Verbs With Too Many Interpretations (Not Advised)*
Classify	Enjoy
Compare	Feel
Contrast	Know
Define	Learn
Demonstrate	Understand
Differentiate	Value
Explain	
Predict	
Recall	
Select	
Verbalize	
Write	

Source: Bastable & Doody, 2008.

Other possible shortcomings in writing objectives that preceptors should be aware of include (adapted from Bastable & Doody, 2008):

- Including more than one expected behavior in one objective. "The nurse will identify signs of possible kidney transplant rejection and the appropriate interventions." This objective calls for both the identifiable signs of rejection and the actions, two distinctively separate behaviors that should not be combined into one.

- Expecting a higher level of performance than the orientee is capable of attaining. "The graduate nurse will recognize indications for a possible biopsy based upon signs of kidney transplant rejection." This is an expectation of a nurse beyond the novice level of performance, might exceed scope of practice, and is inappropriate.

- Including unnecessary or unrelated information in an objective. "Identify possible signs of kidney transplant rejection and the nurse's knowledge of immunosuppressive medications." Though an understanding of immunosuppression is important in the treatment of rejection, it is unrelated to the nurse's recognition of possible signs of rejection. This objective also combines two separate concepts into a single objective; this is not measurable and defies the concepts of writing solid objectives.

- Developing an objective that is vague, for which the behavior is not clear. "The nurse is interested in the signs of rejection for a transplanted kidney." Does "interest in" the topic reflect comprehension of or a need for relevant action/inaction? No.

- Failure to include all components of an objective. "List the signs of kidney transplant rejection." This objective fails to identify the learner, a time frame, or knowledge based upon what information. Correctly stated: "Following participation in the Transplant Core Course, the nurse will be able to identify the signs of kidney transplant rejection."

- The focus is upon the preceptor rather than the preceptee. "The preceptor will demonstrate proper central vein catheter care technique." It is the preceptee who is the focus of the objective and the one who needs to demonstrate proper catheter care technique, not the preceptor.

- Vague statements that do not capture the essence of the objective. "The patient will be prepared for discharge." This might be an appropriate outcome because it is global in nature, but it does not identify the specificity needed for an objective. This fails to identify what the patient needs to know with respect to her or his medical condition, medications, what problems warrant contacting a medical professional for troubleshooting, etc., as would be identified in an objective. This also exemplifies the misuse and confusion about appropriate use of the terms outcome and objective.

Effective Statements of Learning Outcomes:

- Are preceptee-focused rather than preceptor-focused
- Focus on learning as a result of the preceptorship experience, rather than on the precepting activity itself
- Reflect the unit or organization's mission and values
- Are in alignment at the course, program, and unit/institutional levels
- Focus on the important, nontrivial aspects of learning that are important to the stakeholders
- Focus on skills and abilities central to nursing and based on professional standards of excellence
- Are broad enough to encompass important learning activities, but clear and specific enough to be measurable
- Focus on areas of learning that will continue to develop and mature, but can be evaluated in the present

Adapted from Huba & Freed, 2000

Conclusion

The preceptor-preceptee relationship is critical to the success of the teaching-learning experience. The very core of this experience is the thoughtful, careful articulation of objectives, goals, and outcomes that are agreed upon by all involved. Using taxonomies such as those presented in this chapter to construct the framework to guide the experience will enhance the opportunities for success!

References

American Association of Colleges of Nursing (2008). *Executive summary. The essentials of baccalaureate education for professional nursing practice.* Washington, DC: Author.

American Nurses Association (ANA). (2001). *Code of ethics for nurses with interpretive statements.* Silver Spring, MD: Author.

American Nurses Association (ANA) & National Nursing Staff Development Organization (NNSDO). (2010). *Nursing professional development: Scope and standards of practice.* Silver Spring, MD: Author.

Baltimore, J. J. (2004). The hospital clinical preceptor: Essential preparation for success. *The Journal of Continuing Education in Nursing, 35*(3), 133-140.

Bastable, S. B., & Doody, J. A. (2008). Behavioral objectives. In S. B. Bastable (Ed.), *Nurse as Educator* (3rd ed., pp. 383-427). Sudbury, MA: Jones and Bartlett.

Bloom, B. (Ed.). (1956). *Taxonomy of educational objectives, the classification of educational goals—Handbook I: Cognitive domain*, New York: McKay.

Bresciani, M. J. (n.d.). *Writing measurable and meaningful outcomes*. Retrieved from http://www.ncsu.edu/assessment/evaluation/writingoutcomes.pdf

Burns, H. K., & Northcutt, T. (2009). Supporting preceptors: A three-pronged approach for success. *The Journal of Continuing Education in Nursing, 40*(11), 509-513.

Churches, A. (2008). Retrieved from http://teachnology.pbworks.com/f/Bloom%5C%27s+Taxonomy+Blooms+Digitally.pdf

Churches, A. (2009). Retrieved from http://edorigami.wikispaces.com/file/view/bloom%27s+Digital+taxonomy+v3.01.pdf

Davis, K., Chen, Y., & Cambell, M. (2010). Bloom—biography, in Bloom's Taxonomy: Original and revised. In M. Orey (Ed.), *Emerging perspectives on learning, teaching and technology*, (p.7). Retrieved from http://projects.coe.uga.edu/epltt/index.php?title=Bloom%27s_Taxonomy

Duclos-Miller, P. A. (2006). *Stressed out about your first year of nursing*. Marblehead, MA: HCPro, Inc.

Fink, L. D. (2003). *Creating significant learning experiences*. San Francisco, CA: Jossey-Bass.

Forehand, M. (2005). Bloom's Taxonomy: Original and revised. In M. Orey (Ed.), *Emerging perspectives on learning, teaching and technology*. Retrieved from http://projects.coe.uga.edu/epltt/index.php?title=Bloom%27s_Taxonomy

Glennon, C. D. (2006). Reconceptualizing program outcomes. *Journal of Nursing Education, 45*(2), 55-58.

Goleman, D. (1998). *Working with emotional intelligence*. New York: Bantam Books.

Heinich, R., Molenda, M., Russell, J., & Smaldino, S. (2001). *Instructional methods and technologies for learning* (7th ed.). Englewood Cliffs, NJ: Prentice Hall, Inc.

Huba, M., & Freed, J. (2000). Meaningful assessment of intended learning outcomes from learner-centered assessment on college campuses. In *Practical tips for writing measurable outcomes*. UT Health Science Center Academic Center for Excellence in Teaching. Retrieved from www.uthscsa.edu/acet/docs/TFDN/Wuest.doc

Mager, R.F. (1997). *Preparing instructional objectives: A critical tool in the development of effective instruction* (3rd ed.). Atlanta, GA: Center for Effective Performance.

Murphy, B. (2008). Positive precepting: Preparation can reduce the stress. *MEDSURG Nursing, 17*(3), 183-188.

Nesbitt, S. W. (2006). Adult learning concepts. In J. P. Flynn & M. C. Stack (Eds.), *The role of the preceptor: A guide for nurse educators, clinicians and managers* (2nd ed., pp. 15-27). New York, NY: Springer Publishing Company.

Neumann, J. A., & Forsyth, D. (2008). Teaching in the affective domain for institutional values. *The Journal of Continuing Education in Nursing, 39*(6), 248-252.

O'Neill, G., & Murphy, F. (2010). Guidelines to taxonomies of learning. *University College Dublin.* Retrieved from http://www.ucd.ie/t4cms/UCDTLA0034.pdf

Oregon State University. (2011). *Models—Course development. Instructional design—The taxonomy table. How to write objectives.* Retrieved from http://oregonstate.edu/instruct/coursedev/models/id/taxonomy/

Simpson, E. J. (1966-67). The classification of educational objectives, psychomotor domain, *Illinois Teacher of Home Economics, 10,* 110-144. Retrieved from http://epsilonlearning.com/outcomes_taxonomy.pdf

Simpson, E. J. (1972). The classification of educational objectives in the psychomotor domain. In M. T. Rainier (Ed.), *Contributions of behavioral science to instructional technology: The psychomotor domain* (3rd ed.). Englewood Cliffs, NJ: Gryphon Press, Prentice-Hall.

Smedley, A., Morey, P., & Race, P. (2010). Enhancing the knowledge, attitudes, and skills of preceptors: An Australian perspective. *Journal of Continuing Education in Nursing, 41*(10), 451-461.

Su, W. M., Osisek, P. J., & Starnes, B. (2004). Applying the revised Bloom's Taxonomy to medical-surgical nursing lesson. *Nurse Educator, 29*(3), 116-120.

Ullrich, S., & Haffer, A. (2009). *Precepting in nursing: Developing an effective workforce.* Sudbury, MA: Jones and Bartlett Publishers.

University of Central Florida & Seminole Community College (2008). Method for assessing student outcomes: MATURE. In *Practical tips for writing measurable outcomes.* UT Health Science Center Academic Center for Excellence in Teaching. Retrieved from www.uthscsa.edu/acet/docs/TFDN/Wuest.doc

University of Mississippi. (n.d.). *Bloom's taxonomy: Psychomotor domain.* Retrieved from slo.sbcc.edu/wp-content/uploads/blooms-psychomotor-domain4.doc

Waller, K. V. (2001). Writing instructional objectives. *National Accrediting Agency for Clinical Laboratory Services (NAACLS).* Retrieved from www.naacls.org/docs/announcement/writing-objectives.pdf

Wittman-Price, R. A., & Fasolka, B. J., 2010. Objectives and outcomes: The fundamental difference. *Nursing Education Perspective, 31*(4), 233-236.

Preceptor Development Plan
Having a Plan: Developing and Using Objectives, Goals, and Outcomes

Review the information on developing and using objectives, goals, and outcomes described in this chapter. What are your strengths? In which areas do you need to increase your knowledge and expertise? What is your plan for expanding your knowledge and expertise? What resources are available? Who can help you?

Review the overall objectives, goals, and outcomes that are required for your preceptee throughout their onboarding experience. If written descriptions of the objectives, goals, and outcomes are not available, work with other stakeholders to develop them. Based on these objectives, goals, and outcomes, create a plan for your preceptee.

Name:			
Taxonomies of Learning			
Strengths	Needs	Plan	Resources
Developing Goals			
Strengths	Needs	Plan	Resources
Developing Outcomes			
Strengths	Needs	Plan	Resources
Developing Objectives			
Strengths	Needs	Plan	Resources

Note: This form and other resources are available at www.RNPreceptor.com.

Preceptor Development Plan **Having a Plan: Developing and Using Objectives,** **Goals, and Outcomes**		
Role:		
Goal:		
Outcome:		
Objective	Plan of Action	
	Time Frame	Plan
Goal:		
Outcome:		
Objective	Plan of Action	
	Time Frame	Plan
Goal:		
Outcome:		
Objective	Plan of Action	
	Time Frame	Plan

Note: This form and other resources are available at www.RNPreceptor.com.

"Communication works for those who work at it."
–John Powell

Communication

Laurie Shiparski, MS, BSN, RN

6

Communication is something that people have to work on their entire lives. In health care, it has wide-ranging impacts on patient safety and satisfaction, staff satisfaction, and interdisciplinary team effectiveness, and in creating healthy work cultures. Because of this impact, all health care team members must be involved in ongoing, intentional work to improve the communication. It is a critical competency for preceptors and preceptees to master. Improving communication can be an overwhelming topic to explore, considering the plethora of information and research available. This chapter focuses directly on the practical application of five key dialogue skills that form the foundation for effective communication. In addition, this chapter contains an emphasis on preceptor-preceptee communication, the enhancement of team communications, patient safety and handoffs, and strategies for preceptor training/meetings.

The Five Skills of Effective Communication

Preceptors and preceptees can work on improving communication in many ways. Dialogue is one way to focus on communication; it is about creating ways to interact, work, and be together. William Isaacs (1999), who founded the Dialogue Project at MIT's Sloan School of Management, defines *dialogue* as the discipline of collective learning and inquiry—a process for transforming the quality of conversation.

The role of the preceptor is to become an excellent communicator and role model of dialogue and to invite and encourage other

OBJECTIVES

- Describe the five core skills of effective communication for preceptees and preceptors

- Articulate the behaviors for self-improvement of dialogue skills

- Distinguish effective ways of managing different methods of communication

- Name key considerations for participating in team communications

- State ways to manage difficult conversations between preceptors and preceptees

colleagues to do the same. This does not mean that the preceptor is a perfect communicator. You are going to have times when miscommunication occurs or times when an interaction could have been handled better. The important thing is to see effective communication and dialogue as ongoing learning processes. Each interaction should be treated as an opportunity to practice the skills and grow.

The following dialogue beliefs help to frame our interactions:

- Many different ways to think about something exist.

- Each person has innate wisdom.

- As each person sees something different, we all have opportunity to see it more clearly.

- Opposites are connected to the same truths.

- See and welcome the wisdom in the resistance (Wesorick & Shiparski, 1997).

You need to have facility with five key dialogue skills: intent, listening, advocacy, inquiry, and silence. You also need to know what can be gained from using these five skills. The preceptor can practice these skills to create effective communication with preceptees, colleagues, and patients. These five skills can be useful in situations when you:

- Explore an issue.

- Accomplish transformative work.

- Evoke wisdom from individuals and groups.

- Generate new knowledge.

- Create mutual opportunities for healing the workplace, care providers, patients, and families.

- Accelerate breakthrough experiences with issues and challenges (Wesorick & Shiparski, 1997).

Using these five dialogue skills helps you to learn core skills that can provide a foundation for effective communication for individuals and the team. Over the past few decades, these skills have been useful in moving conversations to effective levels in health care and other industries. As a preceptor, leader, and mentor, you will find the skills of intent, listening, advocacy, inquiry, and silence invaluable to being successful in your role.

Intent

The first skill is intent, and it sets the stage for people to connect in healthy ways. Intent involves creating a safe place that invites participation and authenticity. It also refers to the capacity for individuals and teams to connect in mission and purpose and move forward with action. In the preceptor-preceptee relationship, preceptors have the responsibility to state their own intent and then invite preceptees to share their own intent. At the onset of the relationship, preceptors can share their answers to the following intent questions and then invite preceptees to do the same.

- Without being humble, what do you value most about yourself, your work, your organization?

- What are the most important things you would like to get out of this experience?

After answering the two questions, take a moment to offer two to three concrete actions that each of you can take to ensure the preceptor-preceptee relationship will support the intents shared.

Listening

Listening is the second dialogue skill and is one of the most important of all. When you listen to another person, you pay that person the highest respect and honor possible. In the fast-paced day of a preceptor, this skill is at risk of being lost. You need to pause and remind yourself to really listen to those around you. Be fully present.

To practice this skill, consider that listening can occur on four levels: listening to self, to others, to the collective, and between the lines (Wesorick & Shiparski, 1997).

Listening to yourself means noticing the voice in your head and your intuition or gut feeling. When you are in a situation, be aware of the wisdom that your body, mind, and spirit are offering you. This is especially helpful with patient situations and preceptee interactions. If you hear a criticizing voice, then be aware, but don't let it hold you back. If you hear intuition, reveal and act on it if it seems right. Teach the preceptee to do the same.

In listening to others, listen with your heart and head. Be present in the moment.

Listening to the collective refers to listening to the bigger picture of a group conversation. This kind of listening can be applied in talking with a family or group of preceptees or other staff. The preceptor must watch for themes and patterns and then name them for the group. The pattern might require an action to follow up. An example would be if a group of preceptees discussed its experiences on a particular unit and each individual story led to uncovering a pattern that this unit was highly supportive of preceptees. Key behaviors of the unit staff might be enhancing the success of the preceptee experience. The preceptor could then follow up by sharing the positive feedback with the unit named and other units.

Finally, listening between the lines refers to working with a group and noticing that its words and actions don't match. Or, you get a sense that something else is going on in the group that is not being spoken. For example, a preceptor and preceptee were talking about the poor prognosis of a critically ill patient to her children and husband. As they discussed options, the family was very engaged and helpful, but an overriding resistance and anger seemed to be present. The preceptor noticed the pattern and asked family members what the underlying issue of their emotion and concern was. After a moment of silence, the patient's youngest daughter spoke up to reveal that none of the family members felt they could take care of their mother in this state, and they all felt very guilty about even feeling that way. As a result of the preceptor listening between the lines, the family revealed important information.

Advancing listening skills takes effort and practice. Improving listening skills must be an ongoing intentional action. However, the effort is worth it, because you are showing this respect and dignity to other human beings.

Advocacy

What comes to your mind when you hear the word *advocacy*? As a preceptor, you might think of advocating for the needs of patients or advocating for a good learning assignment for your preceptee. This definition usually means you are trying to convince others to support you in your efforts. Dialogue has a different definition for advocacy. It is the willingness to share personal thinking and what is behind the thinking with the intention of exposing, not defending it (Wesorick & Shiparski, 1997). Advocacy requires the courage to speak your truth and check assumptions to avoid making judgments. It is not about convincing others at all.

One of the most useful tools in understanding how this occurs in our communication efforts is the "ladder of inference," which comes from Peter Senge's work (Senge, 1990; see Figure 6.1). Your thoughts can quickly jump up the ladder as you observe the words and actions of others. The rungs of the ladder represent the following sequence of events: First, you see the actions of another. Second, you add your own meaning. Third, you jump to your own conclusions. Finally, you take actions based on it. You are at risk of acting on your assumptions, even if they are wrong. Have you ever jumped up your ladder only to find you were wrong?

For example, a group of preceptees was in an onboarding class, and the topic was about severe wound care. As the instructor went into more graphic description and showed illustrations of severe wounds, one of the preceptees abruptly got up and ran out of the room (the action). The instructor noticed the action and wondered if the information had been too much for the preceptee (he added her meaning). The instructor drew a conclusion—maybe this preceptee is not strong enough to handle sicker patients. Based on her conclusion and belief, the instructor took action and notified the preceptor of the incident. But the instructor jumped to conclusions. She should have used questions to ask the preceptee what had happened. Later the preceptor did ask and found out that the preceptee had not been feeling well that morning and came to work ill. It had nothing to do with her ability to handle the topic.

You can use the ladder of inference in three ways:

1. Becoming more aware of your own thinking and reasoning

2. Making your thinking and reasoning more visible to others

3. Inquiring into the thinking and reasoning of others

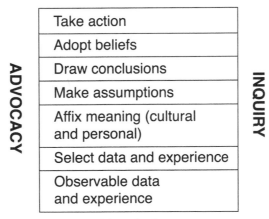

Figure 6.1   The Ladder of Inference (Source: Senge, 1990)

Inquiry

For preceptors, the skill and art of asking questions are invaluable. In dialogue, this is called the skill of inquiry. It is the willingness to ask genuine questions of curiosity to learn from self and others (Wesorick & Shiparski, 1997). On occasion, the preceptor will need to ask questions to see what the preceptee knows and understands. This is part of the learning process. In addition, some questions help preceptees dig deeper to uncover the wisdom that is inside them. Self-realization and discovery make for a powerful learning experience, so rather than just giving the answers to questions, the preceptor can advance questions to evoke deeper learning. The following are examples of different kinds of coaching questions that preceptors can use when trying to understand and deepen learning (Wesorick & Shiparski, 1997).

- What leads you to think that? Give data.
- Could you give me an example?
- Could you say more about that?
- What do you mean by . . . ?
- How do you feel about that?
- I'm asking because . . .

Questions that can be used when trying to broaden thinking include:

- What values might others have that would help us understand this situation or think differently about it?
- What might I/we be missing by looking at the issue from my/our view?

Another type of deeper questioning is called *appreciative inquiry*. It is a methodology developed by David Cooperrider, a professor of organizational behavior at Case Western Reserve University. It is the skill of using a positive, appreciative approach to questioning, and it differs from the traditional approach (Hammond, 1998; see Figure 6.2).

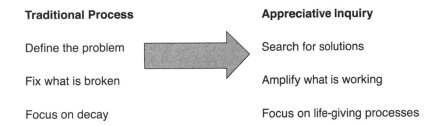

Traditional Process		Appreciative Inquiry
Define the problem		Search for solutions
Fix what is broken		Amplify what is working
Focus on decay		Focus on life-giving processes

Figure 6.2   Traditional Process vs. Appreciative Inquiry

In health care, we tend to focus on fixing the problems and often do not tap this appreciative approach to grow our knowledge of what is working. It is necessary to recognize the problems and to balance that recognition with noticing what works. Preceptors who want to inspire others and teach in energizing ways use this type of questioning. Cooperrider and Whitney (2005) offer the following underlying assumptions of appreciative inquiry:

- In every society, organization, or group, something works.
- What we focus on becomes our reality.
- The act of asking questions of an individual, group, or organization influences them in some way.
- What we want already exists in ourselves, our firms, our organizations, and our communities.

When preceptors communicate with an appreciative approach, they can spark imagination, innovation, and creativity and evoke essential values and learning. Good appreciative questions are stated in the affirmative and are always presented as an invitation to answer them. The following are examples of appreciative inquiry questions that can be used with preceptees:

- What do you like about your experience so far?
- What's working well? What should we keep doing that is working?
- Think back through your career/experience. Locate a moment that was a high point when you felt most effective and engaged. Describe how you felt and what made the situation possible.
- How can we be more supportive of you?

Silence

Silence is the willingness to experience and learn by reflecting and discovering the lessons from personal awareness, words unspoken, or the quiet of the soul (Wesorick & Shiparski, 1997). Good preceptors know the power of this skill. It might happen with patients as you sit quietly at their bedside and support them with your presence, with no words needing to be spoken. Silence can arise when you are sitting with a preceptee who is conveying a heart-moving story about a patient experience.

The skill comes in how you handle silence when it occurs. You have to ask yourself if silence makes you uncomfortable. Those with experience in silence have built a comfort level to be in it calmly and fully when it arises. It represents a profound moment, and you have the potential for many moments in your caring as long as you recognize and welcome it.

In some ways, you can use silence to help in situations. A preceptor can ask a preceptee to leave an intense patient situation for a few minutes to be in silence and regain calm perspective. If in a tense patient-family situation where emotions are running high, the preceptee can call for a few moments of silence for all to regroup. This can de-escalate a situation immediately. In another application of silence, the preceptor can ask the preceptee to be in silence to reflect on the learning that is occurring for them.

Also, at times, preceptors might find a few minutes of silence necessary to regroup or reenergize. A quote from Jiddu Krishnamurti summarizes the power of silence, "Real communication can only take place where there is silence."

Checklist: Dialogue Behaviors for Self

- ❑ Intent
  - ❑ Clarify personal intent and act on it.
  - ❑ Show vulnerability.
  - ❑ Show up authentically.
  - ❑ Respect the wisdom of self and others.
- ❑ Listening
  - ❑ Listen on all levels: self and others, as well as the collective (internal and external).
  - ❑ Hear internal voice, but know how to move beyond negative self-talk, fear, and worry.
  - ❑ Listen with your heart.
  - ❑ Honor self and each other.
- ❑ Advocacy
  - ❑ Speak your truth (be courageous).
  - ❑ Manage candor and diplomacy as an ongoing dynamic.
  - ❑ Share your thoughts and feelings to reveal a perspective, not convince others.
  - ❑ Check out your assumptions.
  - ❑ Avoid judgments of self and others.
- ❑ Inquiry
  - ❑ Ask genuine questions of curiosity to learn from self and others.
  - ❑ Use questions as a personal reflection tool to uncover new perspectives and wisdom.
  - ❑ Utilize questions that help you remember what worked before, questions that grow what is working well, and build on your strengths (appreciative inquiry).
- ❑ Silence
  - ❑ Create space to think and reflect.
  - ❑ Be present in the moment.
  - ❑ Call for silence to de-escalate a situation.

Managing Different Methods of Communication

The skills reviewed thus far are applicable to all forms of verbal, e-mail, texting, and other written communications. Though face-to-face communication is always the best mode, in this age of technology, our interactions often take place via e-mail, texting, or phone. The critical factor to consider when communicating by these latter methods is that the risk of misunderstanding is higher. The possibility of jumping to conclusions is much higher, because you cannot tell the intent or tone of the communication. The following tips for the preceptor can improve the effectiveness of e-mail communication:

- If it is a sensitive or confidential topic, consider calling or meeting in person instead of writing an e-mail. Do not send confidential patient information unless approved by the organization.

- Never write anything in an e-mail that you wouldn't share with anyone.

- Keep messages short. Detail can be shared in person if necessary.

- Check your spelling.

- Use both uppercase and lowercase letters. It is considered rude to write in all caps.

- If you're responding to a message, be aware of the "reply all" option and do not send the response to all if it is not necessary.

- If you're sending an important message, test it by sending it to yourself first.

- Answer your e-mail quickly and avoid not responding, because it can convey a lack of respect.

- If you receive an e-mail that conveys anger or upsets you in any way, follow up and check with the sender in person to clarify intent and message.

In addition, be very cautious of sharing any patient- or work-related information on social networking sites, unless they are internally protected sites within the health care organization.

Patient Safety and Handoffs

Communication is one of the key strategies for ensuring patient safety. Preceptors have a responsibility to discuss the importance of this with preceptees and to offer strategies to help them communicate appropriately. The Institute of Medicine (IOM) has identified that as many as 98,000 annual deaths occur as a result of errors (Kohn, Corrigan, & Donaldson, 2000). The Joint Commission review of sentinel event data consistently finds that communication (or lack of communication) is the number one cause of sentinel events (The Joint Commission, 2011). Many of these errors and sentinel events can be eliminated with effective communication.

Handoffs are a major area that has been identified in which communication can prevent errors and improve patient outcomes. The IOM recommends that handoff communication occur in a verbal mode, where questions and explanations can be exchanged. Currently, many formats that guide communication for patient handoffs exist, and it is believed that a standard approach does increase the effectiveness of the exchange.

One frequently used communication tool is the ISBAR format, which offers key points for communicating during patient handoffs:

I—Introduction

S—Situation (the current issue)

B—Background (brief, related to the point)

A—Assessment (what you found/think)

R—Recommendation/request (what you want next)

The preceptor needs to review what happens in situations when the preceptee feels a patient need is not being addressed. Preceptees must be encouraged to speak up and not hold back because of fear of repercussions from physicians or others. Preceptors can find it helpful, for example, to role-play a situation where a patient is in trouble and it is difficult to get the attention of the physician. Ensure that the preceptee utilizes the dialogue skills and seeks backup help from supervisors and staff mentors. Preceptees should not go it alone in tough clinical situations in which they are not being heard.

The Association of periOperative Registered Nurses (AORN; 2007) has developed a communication checklist for handoffs.

❑ Get the person's attention.

❑ Make eye contact; face the person.

❑ Use the person's name.

❑ Express concern.

❑ Utilize a handoff format such as ISBAR.

❑ Re-assert as necessary.

❑ Decision reached.

❑ Escalate if necessary.

Handoffs are also important when a preceptee is being handed off to another preceptor. Just as with patient handoffs, good communication during a preceptee handoff can help ensure a smooth, efficient transition and maximize outcomes.

Considerations for Participating in Team Communications

Thus far in this chapter, the focus has been on communication skills between preceptor and preceptee and with patients and their families. It is the role of the preceptor to emphasize and discuss ways to interact with the interdisciplinary team as well. Whether in staff meetings, during interdisciplinary rounds, or in care conferences, preceptees have to master the art of team communication to be successful in their role. Tips on participating in team conversations include:

- Be aware that your goal is to contribute in respectful, thoughtful ways.

- Utilize the dialogue skills.

- Be present and attentive—be an observer of the process and what is being said.

- Have the courage to speak your truth and think before you speak it. Present your ideas and comments in calm, diplomatic ways so others can hear them.

- Ask questions to clarify what others are saying and to understand their perspectives without evoking defensiveness. Check your assumptions. One approach could be to say, "That is an interesting perspective. I'd like to understand more about that."

- Encourage others to participate and state your appreciation for the contribution of others.

- Basically, give to others what you would like for them to give to the conversation.

Managing Difficult Conversations

One of the most useful skills to have is the ability to manage difficult conversations. The basis for effective communication in these situations is use of the dialogue skills, but you have a few more strategies. All of us at some time or another bump up against a tough conversation. Many times, we find ourselves avoiding them, and in many cases, this perpetuates strained relationships and de-energizes workplaces. Preceptors should spend time discussing the importance of having these difficult conversations with others in the workplace to address patient issues and interpersonal issues. Deepak Chopra (1997) offers some insight into why these situations arise: "When you struggle with your partner, you are struggling with yourself. Every fault you see in them touches a denied weakness in yourself." The important thing is that we make these conversations happen. A good resource is *Crucial Conversations: Tools for Talking When Stakes Are High* (Patterson, Grenny, McMillian, & Switzler, 2002). Patterson and colleagues describe a process for managing these difficult conversations:

1. Start with your heart. Identify what you really want for yourself, others, and the relationship. How would I behave if I really did want this?

2. Learn to look. Identify it when a conversation is crucial, and identify the risk. Is there stress involved?

3. Make it safe. Apologize, fix misunderstandings, and maintain mutual respect.

4. State your path.

5. Explore others' paths.

6. Agree and move on to actions.

It is always helpful to seek to understand the other person's perspective before sharing your own views and to look for the points of agreement to bridge the gap of the disagreement.

Strategies for Education and Meetings

Also, some communication strategies can enhance effective communication in meetings and educational gatherings. The intent or goal of these situations is to create a place where communication is open, honest, and direct. You will find it helpful to state this as an intent to the group to invite them to participate in this way. One strategy is to take time to develop a list of behaviors that the group can commit to practicing and using. This can be a short process of about 15 minutes and comes from suggestions in the group. Some examples of these group behaviors include:

- Keep confidentiality.

- Respect all views.

- Check assumptions.

- Speak your truth.

- Bring up "undiscussables."

- Assume a positive intent from others.

An agreement to behaviors such as these can lay the foundation to invite everyone to participate safely. Readings (poems, stories, etc.) can be used to set the stage for effective communication (Shiparski, 2002).

Another strategy is utilizing a "check-in" process at the beginning or end of a meeting. This process is used when you want to invite participation, practice dialogue skills, and create an environment of learning and connection. Check-in is when all in attendance get a chance to speak without interruption. It works best when the participants are seated in a circle. The facilitator or leader extends a welcome and introduces the process. Doing a reading or calling for a moment of silence at the beginning of the meeting to get everyone's attention and presence is helpful. Then the facilitator offers a question for each person to answer. Some examples are as follows:

- What is something about you we don't know?

- What's up for you today?

- What did you have to leave behind to be present here?

- What energizes you at work?

- What is most important to you about the topic we are discussing today? (Name the topic.)

Full and Empty

Our meetings are full
of schedules,
timed talk
and quick decisions.

They are full
of words that swirl
at the surface
of deeper issues.

They are full
of giving information,
fixing problems,
and staying on track.

They are full
of ego building,
defending, blaming,
and judgment of others.

They are full
of quieting the voices,
that bring questions and
unwanted truths.

Our meetings are full
and I am left empty.
Our meetings are full
and I am left empty.

Give me one clear
moment of silence
and the courage
to show my vulnerable self.

Let me be an invitation
for us to be together
in a meaningful,
genuine way.

–Laurie Shiparski, 2002

After a question is presented, each person takes a turn around the table to briefly speak his or her answer. This process allows the group to know something more about each individual, and it invites further participation.

Sometimes groups pass an object around the table to slow the process down and indicate when they are done speaking (Shiparski, 2002). Other variations of this strategy exist: One is to do a round robin to hear from each person at the end of a meeting with a one- or two-word description of how each person is feeling.

Conclusion

These practical techniques can help create cultures of effective communication and connection for preceptors, preceptees, and the patients and staff with whom they work. The ongoing, intentional effort invested in learning and practicing these skills can have a significantly positive effect on patient outcomes, interdisciplinary teamwork, and effective teaching and learning experiences. In addition, as you learn to manage your communication and interactions in healthy ways, your stress can be reduced and your effectiveness increased.

References

Association of periOperative Registered Nurses (AORN). (2007). *Handoff standardizing.* Retrieved from www.aorn.org/PracticeResources/ToolKits/PatientHandoffToolKit/

Chopra, D. (1997). An excerpt from *The path to love: Renewing the power of spirit in your life.* Retrieved from http://deepakchopra.wwwhubs.com/chopra6.htm

Cooperrider, D., & Whitney, D. (2005). *Appreciative inquiry: A positive revolution in change.* San Francisco, CA: Berrett-Koehler.

Hammond, S. A. (1998). *The thin book of appreciative inquiry.* Bend, OR: TB Publishing.

Isaacs, W. (1999). *Dialogue and the art of thinking together.* New York, NY: Doubleday.

Kohn, L. T., Corrigan, J. M., & Donaldson, M. S. (Eds.). (2000). *To err is human: Building a safer health system.* Washington, DC: National Academy Press.

Patterson, K., Grenny, J., McMillian, R., & Switzler, A. (2002). *Crucial conversations: Tools for talking when stakes are high.* New York, NY: McGraw-Hill.

Senge, P. (1990). *The fifth discipline: The art & practice of the learning organization.* New York, NY: Doubleday.

Shiparski, L. (2002). *Turning points: A dialogue tool for realizing personal and group wisdom.* Grand Rapids, MI: Practice Field Publishing.

The Joint Commission. (2011). *Collation of sentinel event-related data reported to The Joint Commission (1995-2010).* Retrieved from http://www.jointcommission.org/SentinelEvents/Statistics/

Wesorick, B., & Shiparski, L. (1997). *Can the human being thrive in the work place? Dialogue as a strategy of hope.* Grand Rapids, MI: Practice Field Publishing.

Additional Resources

Bohm, D. (2003). *On dialogue* (1st ed.). New York, NY: Routeledge Publishers.

Ellinor, L., & Gerard, G. (1998). *Dialogue: Rediscovering the transformative power of conversation.* Hoboken. NJ: John Wiley & Sons.

Emerald, D. (2005). *The power of TED: The empowerment dynamic.* Bainbridge Island, WA: Polaris Publishing.

Markova, D. (1991). *The art of the possible: A compassionate approach to understanding the way people think, learn and communicate.* Newburyport, MA: Conari Press.

Mendele, A. (1995). *Sitting in the fire: Large group transformation using conflict and diversity.* Portland, OR: Lao Tse Press.

Senge, P., Scharmer, C. O., Jaworski J., & Flowers, B. S. (2004). *Presence: Human purpose and the field of the future.* New York, NY: Doubleday.

Whitney, D., Cooperrider, D. L., Trosten-Bloom, A., & Kaplan, B. S. (2001). *Encyclopedia of Positive Questions Volume 1: Using appreciative inquiry to bring out the best in your organization.* Brunswick, OH: Crown Custom Publishing.

Yankelovich, D. (1999). *The magic of dialogue: Transforming conflict into cooperation.* Austin, TX: Touchstone Publishing.

Preceptor Development Plan
Communication

Review the information on communication described in this chapter. What are your strengths? In which areas do you need to increase your knowledge and expertise? What is your plan for expanding your knowledge and expertise? What resources are available? Who can help you?

Name:			
Intent			
Strengths	Needs	Plan	Resources
Listening			
Strengths	Needs	Plan	Resources
Advocacy			
Strengths	Needs	Plan	Resources
Silence			
Strengths	Needs	Plan	Resources
Handoffs			
Strengths	Needs	Plan	Resources
Team Communications			
Strengths	Needs	Plan	Resources
Difficult Conversations			
Strengths	Needs	Plan	Resources

Note: This form and other resources are available at www.RNPreceptor.com.

"You cannot teach a man anything; you can only help him find it within himself."

–Galileo

Coaching

Laurie Shiparski, MS, BSN, RN

Coaching is about helping others find the answers within themselves, gain understanding and meaning in their circumstances, and take action to move through their challenges. The most effective preceptors are those who can enter into a coaching relationship with their preceptees. This chapter contains valuable information on the role of a coach, ways to develop and conduct a coaching relationship, and coaching techniques that inspire others to tap their own wisdom, passion, perseverance, and strength.

What Is the Role of the Preceptor as Coach?

Every preceptor has the capacity to be a coach. When we support ourselves or others in personal and professional growth, we are coaching. When we assist others in problem solving, learning, and transitioning, we are coaching. Preceptors often find themselves in a role of encouraging others, inspiring others to take on new challenges, and taking action for change. This is all coaching. It is a skill and an art that requires the use of tools and processes as well as relationship development. Each coaching relationship and interaction is a unique connection.

To be an effective coach, the preceptor must possess some foundational behaviors and beliefs which guide the learning process and outcomes. Coaching behaviors and beliefs include:

- Each preceptee has wisdom and the capacity for learning.

OBJECTIVES

- Describe the role of the preceptor as coach

- Identify ways to set up a coaching agreement and utilize a coaching interaction format with preceptees

- Articulate strategies to inspire learning and move through challenges

- Identify the preceptor's role in working with resistance and edges

- Describe how a preceptor ends a coaching relationship with a preceptee

- Coaching is a skill and an art.

- All of our experiences and parts of ourselves are necessary and make us who we are today.

- Each of us is unique and on our own journey of learning and self-awareness. The preceptor has to meet the preceptee where the preceptee is in that journey.

- What goes on inside each of us is as important as what is happening outside of us.

- Coaching addresses the health of body, mind, and spirit in both our work and personal lives. We are whole people, and all our aspects are connected.

- What we resist persists. If we focus only on learners' deficits, they will not grow.

- Conflict is normal and essential to growth. Preceptors need to expect it and find the wisdom in the resistance.

- All problems and challenges are our teachers; they offer opportunities for growth.

- Focusing on the preceptee's strengths and new possibilities is far more motivating than identifying everything that is going wrong.

- Preceptors do not just give all the answers, but use questions and observations to evoke the preceptee's own awareness and wisdom.

With these beliefs and behaviors in mind, the preceptor can make meaning of situations that arise as the relationship and learning unfold. No matter what level of frustration, stuckness, or emotion arises in the preceptee, the role of the preceptor is to be calm and use every situation as a learning opportunity.

Setting Up a Coaching Agreement With a Preceptee

You need to establish coaching agreements and boundaries at the onset of the relationship. The preceptor initiates this discussion with the preceptee and finalizes the agreement. The preceptor first describes what the role of a coach entails, offers times and places for meetings with the preceptee, and clarifies the expectation that both parties will honor the agreements and respect each other's roles. It is imperative that a conversation happen in which the preceptor offers what he or she brings to the relationship and what is needed from the preceptee for optimal learning and support. In turn, the preceptee then gets a chance to express what he or she needs from the preceptor and explains what he or she is willing to give in order to make the relationship effective. The following represents a few examples of these mutual agreements.

We will:

- Have open, direct communication
- Respect each other's opinions and viewpoints
- Keep confidences as part of building our trust
- Listen intently to each other
- Check our assumptions
- Avoid judgment and jumping to conclusions
- Honor each other by beginning and ending our meeting times as planned or discussed
- Seek to understand each other and assume positive intent in all actions
- Forgive and move on as challenges arise

Preceptors can achieve greater levels of engagement if they enter into coaching relationships by staying as impartial as possible. This means they have to own and be upfront about their own judgments and biases. Preceptors have to be open to diverse views and let the preceptees be responsible for fueling their own processes, making choices, and mutually determining outcomes.

Utilizing a Coaching Interaction Format

When conducting a coaching interaction, you will find it helpful to have a format and questions to guide the process. One option is called 4 Gateways Coaching (Daly, 2007; see Table 7.1). This four-step process ensures a clear understanding of an issue and the actions to move through it. You need to take notes during the session, and the format provides a sample worksheet to guide the interaction and document next steps. This four-step process does take some time, so plan 45–60 minutes for the coaching interaction. Another way preceptors can use 4 Gateways Coaching is to become comfortable with the questions and utilize them in teaching moments.

Table 7.1 4 Gateways Coaching Process
1. Clarify the issue and desired outcome.
2. Address the issue from four perspectives: thinking, feeling, doing, knowing.
3. Integrate the learning.
4. Identify actions and support.

The first step of 4 Gateways Coaching is to identify the issue at hand. Often an issue arises that needs to be addressed, or it could be that the preceptee issue is unknown and the preceptor has to question and help identify it. The preceptor can do this by asking the preceptee questions such as:

- How has your day gone?

- What issues are you grappling with now?

- Has anything happened that you feel proud about accomplishing?

- What's on your mind?

- What is going well for you?

If possible, try to get the preceptee to identify a desired outcome of working through the issue.

Second, begin asking questions that help the preceptee gain insights and clarity on the issue. The 4 Gateways Coaching questions are designed to offer a balanced approach to tapping the wisdom of the preceptee. Even though the questions do provide a format, they are not meant to impede additional questions that the preceptor identifies as the process unfolds. As a coach, the preceptor should always be aware of his or her own intuition and insights to be added to the process. The suggested questions for this phase include:

- What are your perceptions and judgments about the situation? Do you see a pattern with this kind of situation?

- How has this pattern or situation served you? What hard truths need to be spoken? What boundaries need to be set?

- How do you feel when you look at yourself in this situation?

- What kind of appreciation or support is needed for you in this situation? How could this be a learning experience? What purpose might it have in your life right now?

Third, the integration of learning from the session should occur. It takes approximately one-fourth of the total coaching time to accomplish this phase. This is the time in which the preceptor assesses how, when, and where to bring the insights of the session into daily life. This is also when the preceptor helps the preceptee integrate the preceptee's internal thinking and external experience. The key questions here are:

- What are your takeaways from this process?

- How would support look?

- Are you willing to take a risk?

- Who would like to see you succeed?

The final phase is identifying action steps and support. The preceptor might have noted action steps the preceptee spoke of during the session that can now be brought up and discussed. Or, the preceptor can ask the preceptee what the logical steps to take for resolution would be. It is completely acceptable for the preceptor to suggest actions to be taken, but critical that the preceptor check to see if the preceptee feels the actions would work for him or her. The preceptee is the one who commits to the action. The preceptor also assures the preceptee that he or she will offer support and check in to see what progress is being made with the action steps. Identifying a time frame for the action steps is very helpful as it creates accountability to the action.

The preceptor can use the Coaching Worksheet as a guide and place for taking notes. The preceptor might want to give the notes to the preceptee for further reflection and thinking on the situation. A sample Coaching Worksheet is shown in Table 7.2.

Table 7.2 Sample Coaching Worksheet (Adapted from Daly, 2007)

Clarify the issue and desired outcome.

Address the issue from four perspectives: thinking, feeling, doing, and knowing.

Even though you are asking several questions, the preceptee does not have to answer each one. As the preceptor, you can pick and choose questions or ask them to provoke thinking. If time is short, conduct only one round of questions.

Sample Questions

- What are your perceptions and judgments about the situation? Do you see a pattern with this kind of situation?

- How has this pattern or situation served you? What hard truths need to be spoken? What boundaries need to be set?

Table 7.2   Sample Coaching Worksheet (cont.)

- How do you feel when you look at yourself in this situation?
- What kind of appreciation or support is needed for you in this situation? How could this be a learning experience? What purpose might it have in your life right now?

Integrate the learning

- What are your takeaways from this process?
- What options are there to consider?
- Are you willing to take a risk?
- Who would like to see you succeed?

Identify actions and support

- What action is worth taking? Identify next steps and time frames. Make sure at least one of the steps can be taken within a couple of days.
- Identify who else can support the preceptee and how the preceptor can support the preceptee. The preceptor should schedule a time to check in with the preceptee on progress made and barriers that might be holding the preceptee back.

A Case Study to Exemplify 4 Gateways Coaching

The following case study shows how one preceptor and preceptee utilized this process to move through an issue. Deb was a new graduate nurse working on a cardiac step-down unit. Her preceptor was Jim, an experienced nurse who had been precepting others for 7 years. An issue surfaced regarding the way that Deb was interacting with physicians about the needs of her patients. Some complaints had surfaced from physicians on the unit because they were not getting notified of patient condition changes in a timely manner. Also, Jim noticed that critical lab results were not being called to physicians in a timely manner. Jim wanted to really get to the bottom of this situation with Deb through a coaching interaction, so they scheduled 45 minutes in a private conference room to talk about it. Jim began the session by sharing the physician feedback and his observations. He then invited Deb to walk through this coaching process, so they both could understand the situation better and identify next steps to move through the challenge. Here are the notes and information from the session:

1. Clarify the issue and desired outcome. Deb identified that she was having difficulty finding the courage to call physicians with patient issues. The outcome she hoped for was to feel confident in knowing what to call physicians about and when.

2. Address the issue from four perspectives.

   a. What are your perceptions and judgments about the situation? Do you see a pattern with this kind of situation? Deb offered that she sometimes saw physicians express anger at other nurses when they called in patient information. She offered that she had noticed a pattern in the past where she had a difficult time bringing information to authority figures such as parents, bosses, and teachers. Her judgment of herself is that she is a bad nurse for not being able to do this part of her job.

   b. How has this pattern or situation served you? What hard truths need to be spoken? What boundaries need to be set? She offered a hard truth in that she saw the risk to patient care if she did not find a way to convey the information to physicians. She also saw that her credibility was taking a hit by not acting on this. Deb shared that, in the past, avoiding confrontation with authority figures had served her in that she had not experienced criticism from them. Another hard truth was that she realized this information was different, and that she had to contact physicians to address patient conditions. Avoidance was not going to work in this situation. The boundaries discussed were about healthy communication with those in authority. Jim reassured her that in speaking with physicians, she would be supported and would not have to endure inappropriate behavior.

   c. How do you feel when you look at yourself in this situation? Deb: "I feel afraid and unsure of myself—afraid my patients' needs aren't being met and afraid to bother the physicians with things that don't matter. My reputation is on the line." Deb began to cry at this point; her emotions were very high regarding this issue. Jim gave her support and time to really feel her fear and sadness. Jim also affirmed that this was a tough situation, but that he believed she could get through it. He also affirmed the deep caring and commitment to her work and patients that he saw in her. The reason she was so emotional was because this was so important, and she really wanted to do the right thing.

   d. What kind of appreciation or support is needed for you in this situation? How could this be a learning experience? What purpose might it have in your life right now? Deb: "I think I am being called to step into my own power as an advocate for patients. I feel this situation is asking me to be courageous, and as

I move through this hurdle, I will gain more self-confidence." She also realized she was learning to have healthy relationships and communication, and that this physician interaction would give her practice. Jim pointed out to Deb that she needed to appreciate her own struggle with this situation, and that many staff members had also dealt with it. She had many peers who will support her.

3. Integrate the learning.

   • What are your takeaways from this process? Deb shared that she realized she had been carrying the stress of not facing this situation, ignoring it in the hope that it would go away. It was clear to her that she had to take the next step and tap the support of those around her. She knew she could do it, now that it was out in the open.

   • What options are there to consider? Deb articulated that she would work with Jim to identify the information to communicate to the physicians and would like to role-play with him about how she would communicate it.

   • Are you willing to take a risk? Who would like to see you succeed? Deb responded that she was willing to take a risk with the support she had. She knew her patients, peers, and even the physicians would want to see her be successful.

4. Identify actions and support. What action is worth taking? Identify next steps and time frames.

   • Jim and Deb decided they would review her four patients today and discuss appropriate information to be called to physicians.

   • Deb will role-play with Jim how to share the information today.

   • Jim also noted three other staff RNs—Cindy, Kyle, and Pete—who were well respected by physicians and were very experienced nurses. Jim would ask them today if Deb can seek out help from them on physician communication.

   • Jim offered tips on how to invite healthy communication and relationships with physicians. He also encouraged Deb to ask the other identified staff for tips.

   • Deb agreed to set up times this week to ask the identified staff members for tips.

   • Jim offered to focus on supporting her to move through this challenge during the remaining time of her orientation.

- Jim also suggested that, in the future, Deb could always seek out his support and the support of the department director if an inappropriate physician interaction occurs.

Strategies to Inspire Learning and Move Through Challenges

In addition to the 4 Gateways Coaching process, preceptors can use other strategies in coaching preceptees and their peers. Often, preceptors are also sought out by other staff for support and advice. When working with a preceptee or peer, the following guidelines are effective for peer coaching. This process can be done in as little as 20 minutes.

- Listen intently to others with your heart and head; give them a chance to explain their situation before offering advice.

- Clarify what you are hearing by saying, "I heard you say_____. Is that right?"

- Break down the parts of what they are grappling with into manageable issues; help them prioritize and address them one at a time. Brainstorm options with them.

- Offer support and empathy; let them know they are not alone in dealing with the issues, and that you believe they can make it through the situation.

- Help them identify three to four steps they can take to begin to move through the situation. For example, if a preceptee or peer is feeling overwhelmed in a situation, you might hear, "I am having a really bad day. There are so many things going wrong. I don't know where to start." You can then offer to listen to what is happening, but tell the individual that you are only going to spend 5–10 minutes on what is happening, so you can move on to brainstorming what can be done about it.

Another strategy is to use a strengths-based and appreciative approach when offering support to others. A strengths-based approach includes noticing and revealing the strengths you see in others that can help them move through their challenges. Often, we are so focused on what we don't have that we forget to recognize what we do have as strengths. For example, if someone is struggling with an overwhelming day, the preceptor might reveal a strength he or she has noticed in that person that can be helpful. The preceptor could say, "Jane, I have noticed you are a very organized person and have a gift for prioritizing what needs to be done. Let's tap that strength of yours to help you get through this day."

Another strategy is to use appreciative inquiry to help the person identify next steps. Appreciative inquiry is a technique that many coaches use to highlight what is working. This methodology was developed by David Cooperrider, a professor of organizational behavior at Case Western Reserve University. In health care, we are conditioned to focus on fixing problems; this is useful, but not enough. Sue Hammond (1998) notes that appreciative inquiry involves searching for solutions, amplifying what is working, and focusing on life-giving processes.

To use appreciative inquiry, preceptors can employ some version of the following questions in any situation (Whitney, Cooperrider, Trosten-Bloom, & Kaplan, 2001).

1. What do you like about what's going on? What's working? Tell me about a time . . .

2. What would you like to have more of? What would you like to do differently? What made that experience so exciting, meaningful, satisfying . . .?

3. How can I help? What do you need from me? How can I support you? What training, resources, etc., can I provide to help you succeed?

The Preceptor's Role in Working With Resistance and Edges

In almost every coaching process, some resistance shows up. Preceptees and peers eventually come to a point at which they have difficulty moving into unfamiliar territory that tests the limits of their experience, and they will not proceed without assessment of the risks. This unfamiliar territory is called their "edge" (Daly, 2007). Often, a preceptee cannot move through an edge without assistance, and the preceptor can be the catalyst to help. The preceptor must be comfortable with conflict and see resistance as an ally that can be helpful in reaching an effective solution. Resistance is not a problem to solve, but rather a dynamic to manage. If a preceptor is not comfortable with resistance and tries to fight or ignore it, it will grow stronger and potentially sabotage the coaching process.

Resistance has always been in our lives, and it is a natural, normal, useful part of us. Each one of us has a risk manager inside of us whose job is to resist change. This internal risk manager has been our protector when change threatens our status quo. When you are working with resistance and edges, the key is to get the preceptee to name the edge, honor it, and work with it. An edge is simply a challenge or dilemma that represents unknown territory for a person to move through. This kind of work is often a deep, insightful process. If the preceptor can help the preceptee name the edge without judgment, that is a great beginning. As a coach, it is imperative to curb your instinct to fix the situation and rely on having the preceptee decide to move through it.

An Edge Story

An example of such an edge came from a coaching interaction between Phil, a preceptor, and Mary, a preceptee. Phil had selected a patient assignment for Mary that was very challenging. He knew it would be a difficult, but excellent, learning experience for her. The patient was a young trauma victim who had a head injury and a poor prognosis for recovery. Mary immediately reacted to the assignment with negativity. She said, "I feel it is unfair that I have this patient. I am not ready for this level of patient. I can't do it, and I am angry that I am put in this situation." She was angry with Phil. Edges often manifest emotions toward the preceptor. This is a sure sign of an edge. The important thing here is for the preceptor to remain calm and *not* engage in the emotion. So Phil began to try and understand where Mary's emotion was coming from and help her name her edge. Initially, the resistance seemed to come from her doubting her abilities, but as Phil questioned her, the real reason became clear. Mary had lost her 17-year-old brother in a motorcycle accident 5 years earlier. In this case, Phil had used four questions to get at the edge (Shiparski, 2002).

1. What leads me to think and act as I do?

2. What is at risk here?

3. Have you ever felt this way before?

4. If this had a purpose, what would it be?

Mary finally realized that this patient triggered her emotions of that event when Phil asked the third question, "Have you ever felt this way before?" She began to cry and release all of her anger and sadness. Phil respectfully sat with Mary and, when his intuition told him the time was right, he offered compassion and understanding. He then asked her what options she saw to be more effective in moving through this edge. He also asked what support she would need to move forward. Mary ultimately decided she could take care of this patient with Phil's help.

Ending a Coaching Relationship With a Preceptee

At the conclusion of an assignment, the preceptor needs to end the relationship as it has been set up and launch the preceptee into the next phase of his or her journey. This is a time to celebrate successes, offer appreciation and encouragement, and let go. The preceptor should plan a concluding celebration meeting with the preceptee. In this meeting, the following topics can be covered:

- Welcome the preceptee to the celebration meeting.

- Review the progress, accomplishments, and strengths of the preceptee. This could include letters of recognition and encouragement from peers and leaders of the department.

- Make this time a checkpoint for both the preceptor and preceptee to reveal their key learning from the relationship. Each exchanges what he or she most appreciated about the other.

- The preceptor as coach reviews supports that are available to the preceptee from here forward.

The power of appreciation fuels the motivation of the preceptee and the preceptor to continue on with confidence and energy. The coaching relationship should always have mutual learning and benefit for both parties. It is crucial that this concluding meeting offer time for each to express gratitude, learning, and well wishes for each other.

Preceptors need to take time at the end of a coaching relationship to reflect on the experience themselves. As a post-relationship checklist, preceptors as coaches should ask themselves these four questions (Daly, 2007):

1. Was I really of service to my preceptee or peer?

2. Did I keep an open mind?

3. How did I feel about myself, my preceptee, and the experience as a whole?

4. Did I trust my own knowing and respect myself and the preceptee?

Conclusion

In conclusion, though approaches and tools are available, the most important things for the preceptor to remember in creating an effective coaching relationship are to be present and aware, listen to your intuition for guidance, and see the learning in all situations. The goal for preceptors using coaching techniques is to create effective teaching-learning experiences and inspire others to tap their own wisdom, passion, perseverance, and strength. Preceptors who use coaching techniques have a distinct advantage in supporting others.

References

Daly, T. (2007). *4 Gateways Coaching: Evoking soul wisdom.* Boulder, CO: Living Arts Publishing.

Hammond, S. (1998). *The thin book of appreciative inquiry.* Bend, OR: TB Publishing.

Shiparski, L. (2002). *Turning points: A dialogue tool for realizing personal and group wisdom.* Grand Rapids, MI: Practice Field Publishing.

Whitney, D., Cooperrider, D. L., Trosten-Bloom, A., & Kaplan, B. S. (2001). *Encyclopedia of positive questions volume 1: Using appreciative inquiry to bring out the best in your organization.* Brunswick, OH: Crown Custom Publishing.

Additional Resources

Flaherty, J. (1999). *Coaching: Evoking excellence in others.* Boston, MA: Butterworth-Heinemann.

Goldsmith, M., & Lyons, L. S. (Eds.) (2006). *Coaching for leadership: The practice of leadership coaching from the world's greatest coaches* (2nd ed.). San Francisco, CA: Pfeiffer.

Hargrove, R. L. (1998). *Masterful coaching: Extraordinary results by impacting people and the way they think and work together.* San Francisco, CA: Pfeiffer.

Sinetar, M. (1998). *The mentor's spirit: Life lessons on leadership and the art of encouragement.* New York, NY: Saint Martins Griffith.

| Preceptor Development Plan |
| Coaching |

Review the information on coaching described in this chapter. What are your strengths? In which areas do you need to increase your knowledge and expertise? What is your plan for expanding your knowledge and expertise? What resources are available? Who can help you?

Name:			
Setting Up a Coaching Agreement			
Strengths	Needs	Plan	Resources
Coaching Process			
Strengths	Needs	Plan	Resources
Inspiring Learning and Moving through Challenges			
Strengths	Needs	Plan	Resources
Working with Resistance and Edges			
Strengths	Needs	Plan	Resources
Ending a Coaching Relationship			
Strengths	Needs	Plan	Resources

Note: This form and other resources are available at www.RNPreceptor.com.

"The only source of knowledge is experience."
–Albert Einstein

Effectively Using Instructional Technologies

8

Cathleen M. Deckers, EdD, RN
Thomas J. Doyle, MSN, RN
Wendy Jo Wilkinson, MSN, ARNP

Today's burgeoning technological capacity, coupled with a new generation of learners who have a high level of digital literacy, mandates that preceptors understand the function and use of instructional technologies; the role these technologies can play as resources for preceptors and preceptees; and how to integrate these technologies into current practice to improve the efficiency, effectiveness, and safety of competency development and validation. This chapter explores some of the newer technological tools and their capabilities for use in onboarding, competency development, and validation and highlights the importance of matching the technology to meet the needs of learners/preceptees.

OBJECTIVES

- Identify the various forms of instructional technology and appropriate uses of each

- Develop a better understanding of the benefits of using high-fidelity patient simulation to facilitate learning and understanding during new-hire and new-specialty orientation

- Identify trends and future uses of instructional technology methodologies

E-Learning

Clark and Mayer (2007) define E-learning as "instruction delivered on a computer by way of CD-ROM, Internet, or intranet with the following features:

- Includes content relevant to the learning objective;

- Uses instructional methods such as examples and practice to help learning;

- Uses media elements such as words and pictures to deliver the content and methods;

- May be instructor-led (synchronous E-learning) or designed for self-paced individual study (asynchronous E-learning);

- Builds new knowledge and skills linked to individual learning goals or to improved organizational performance" (p. 10).

E-learning experiences offer health care educators and preceptors a vehicle to maximize adult learning by delivering knowledge of standards and culture within an easily accessed format. E-learning provides training that maximizes the ability for the pace of learning to be individualized for each participant, which is an attractive feature for the adult learner. The E-learning experience needs to be interactive and participatory to provide learners/preceptees with relevant knowledge that can be used for practical purposes. The experience should provide practice with feedback, tailored instruction, and application of knowledge rather than be a re-creation of the traditional talk-and-test model of teaching.

Several nursing professional organizations have translated specialty orientation and training materials into an online learning format. The American Association of Critical-Care Nurses (AACN) created the *Essentials of Critical Care Orientation* (*ECCO*), which is designed to deliver context-based didactic material that is relevant to the practice setting. The design of the modules is learner-centered and problem-based, providing core concepts and case studies to develop knowledge. These modules are set within a community of practice of expert critical care practitioners to provide nuanced and supplemental feedback important for learning new knowledge within a profession. The goal in developing the modules was to provide an opportunity to build knowledge that created behavioral change in the clinical setting. Application of newly formed decision-making skills and improved confidence are outcomes of this learning program. These modules are now commonly used to drive onboarding to the critical care specialty.

The American Heart Association has translated its didactic preparation for Basic Life Support/Advanced Cardiac Life Support (BLS/ACLS) training into a game-based simulation to provide efficiency in recertification of these essential clinical skills. These E-learning courses provide learners with clinical scenarios in which they must provide the correct life support interventions to match the situation. Feedback loops are customized based on learner responses to provide continuing educational support when and where the individual learner needs it. Upon completion of the online module, the learner is deemed to have attained a baseline level of resuscitation skills and can then schedule a "live" demonstration. The result is an increased level of proficiency in skill demonstration and an efficient use of time for both the learner and instructor.

An example of a web-based program is eDose, a program that provides an authentic environment for mastery of the competencies involved in safe medication administration and is used for assessing nursing students and experienced nurses. These competencies focus on three areas: conception of the dosage calculation, mathematical competencies, and technical competencies. Conceptual competency simply means the learner can translate what has been ordered for the patient versus what is available for administration and can correctly set up the calculation. Mathematical competency centers on the ability to correctly calculate the dose. Finally, technical competency involves translating the dosage calculated into proper and correct administration of the drug to the patient. Based upon constructive learning theory, scaffolding is used to build the numeracy skills of the learner for safe medication administration. The basic tenets of scaffolding assume that new knowledge builds using an existing framework that is modified by and through experience. eDose creates learning scenarios that actively utilize existing information regarding medication administration while introducing new concepts to improve calculation ability. Concepts are introduced starting with simplistic situations and gradually build into more complex concepts as learners build their knowledge base. e-Dose assessments guide learners toward demonstrating mastery in medication administration competency.

Though E-learning provides an important adjunct to training, it does not take the place of clinical learning. If constructed well, E-learning provides a venue for safe practice and acquisition of baseline skills that translate into core performance behaviors in the clinical setting. Online learning provides a venue for safe practice and acquisition of core knowledge that can then be developed through experiential practice with the preceptor in the clinical setting or the simulation lab.

Web-Based Collaboration Tools

Interaction and learning are not confined to the classroom space. Informal learning through peer-to-peer interaction, synthesis, and reflection can comprise a greater share of learners' time than learning in formal settings (Oblinger & Oblinger, 2005). Creation of spaces and activities to engage in opportunities for learning is a new concept for health care educators and preceptors to consider. The software tools of wikis, blogs/vlogs, and podcasts provide new systems to deliver information. The ease of use and wide availability through open source venues have increased their use over the past 10 years. These tools offer a way to enhance and deepen a clinician's learning experiences by providing information sharing, collaboration, and mobility features.

- **Wiki**—A wiki is a collaborative website where content can be created and edited. It is used as a source for obtaining and/or creating knowledge through asynchronous participation of multiple users. It features easy editing, evidence-based referencing, and a venue to construct knowledge collaboratively. It is used as an asynchronous tool that allows groups to gather for cognitive reflection and construction of meaning through a self-defined database (Boulos, Maramba, & Wheeler, 2006). Wikipedia is perhaps the most commonly known wiki site (*www.wikipedia.com*).

- **Blog/Vlog**—A blog functions as an online journal containing information in reverse chronological order about a particular topic. A blog is usually written by one person sharing a perspective about an identified topic, but its creation can be shared among a group. Standard features of blogging software minimally include the ability to post information and pictures and to provide links to articles/videos. Blogs create a dialogue among dispersed individuals by inviting commentary and debate over the knowledge and reflections that are shared within the site. Search features for archived posts and RSS (really simple syndication) feeds are available to keep the user intimately connected with the author's views and updates. Vlogs are mutations of blogs that are created using video modalities.

- **Podcast**—A podcast is an audio file that can be downloaded to a computer or portable MP3/MP4 device to take information "on the go." The feature of mobility is increasingly attractive for learning as busy professionals increase their attempts to multitask to meet the needs of their hectic and full schedules. Health care school curricula readily use this technology to provide recordings of lectures, audiotapes of sample physical assessment sounds, and patient education scripts. iTunes University (iTunes U) would be an example of this type of interface.

Effectiveness of Web-Based Collaboration Tools

The effectiveness of using web-based collaboration tools as learning venues is dependent upon their planned and systematic deployment. Social networking tools are best suited for environments in which dynamic and collaborative learning takes place. Users must be comfortable with negotiating meaning within a larger community of practice. Adaptation, flexibility, and consensus—rather than perfection—are the skills that are practiced within communities of learners using these tools. Learning becomes an evolutionary experience changed and negotiated by the community of practice of experts and novices. These tools allow learners to test their understanding of new knowledge from the periphery, starting out by watching and absorbing the information and transitioning to full participation within the community. Preceptors provide the expert knowledge within these communities of practice, handing down their sage advice and experience to shape the ideas and knowledge base of preceptees. Preceptees, on the other hand, provide new perspectives that in turn can create an improvement of practice for the expert practitioner (Lave & Wenger, 1991). These are the transitions of practice that can be maximized through the use of collaborative tools to capture, highlight, and augment learning in the clinical space.

Simulation

Simulation is a technique used to safely recreate the real world—with or without sophisticated technology—to educate, train, assess performance, probe systems, or conduct research. It dates back at least to early Rome where, to prepare for war, soldiers practiced sword strokes on tree trunks. As their skills improved, they advanced from honing their sword skills on foot to practicing aboard boats and, eventually, on horseback. The Romans also noticed that the warriors were "getting into it more and practicing harder" (Gravenstein, personal communication, February 2000) when the tree trunk was attired in the dress of the enemy, a concept today's experts in simulation refer to as "suspension of disbelief."

Simulation has been used in health care for hundreds of years. Older nurses remember using oranges to practice intramuscular injections and hot dogs to practice dermal injections in the days before injection pads. The use of cadavers to teach gross anatomy can also be a form of simulation.

The Pursuit of Fidelity

Fidelity of simulation is the accuracy of a representation when compared to the real world or the degree to which a representation is similar in a measurable or perceivable manner to a real-world object, feature, or condition. The term *fidelity* also refers to complexity and the ability to recreate reality. In simple words, how real is it?

Fidelity of simulation is measured in three general categories: equipment, environmental, and psychological (see Table 8.1). In health care education and training, *equipment fidelity* refers to how closely a simulator resembles the human body. A body part, such as an arm, is considered low fidelity. A complete, model-driven human mannequin is considered high fidelity. *Environmental fidelity* refers to how closely the location where simulation takes place mimics the real clinical care setting, be it a home environment, clinic, hospital emergency department, operating room, or ICU. *Psychological fidelity* refers to how closely, as perceived by the learner, a simulation approximates the reality of practice; in other words, how "real" it seems (Doyle, 2011a).

Table 8.1   Comparing Simulation Fidelity

Type of simulation	Equipment fidelity	Environmental fidelity	Psychological fidelity
Case studies/role-plays	Low	Low	Low to medium
Partial-task trainers	Medium	Low	Medium
Full-mission or integrated simulators, instructor-driven	Medium	Medium to high	High
Full mission or integrated simulators, model-driven	High	Medium to high	High

Source: Doyle, 2011a. Used with permission.

The various forms of simulation can be viewed as a continuum with regard to fidelity, with partial and complex task trainers as the lowest and integrated simulators the highest:

- Partial and complex task trainers

- Role-play

- Games

- Computer-assisted instruction

- Standardized patients

- Virtual reality and haptic-based systems

- Integrated simulators: low- through high-fidelity simulators (instructor-driven and model-driven) (Nehring, 2010, p. 8).

Partial and complex task trainers—Partial task trainers are models that simulate a subset of physiologic function and might incorporate both normal and abnormal anatomy. Examples of partial task trainers include such current-day simulators as IV arms or urinary catheterization models. It's interesting to note, however, that the first task trainer was a life-size mannequin called "Mrs. Chase." Designed by a nurse who served as superintendent of the Hartford Hospital School of Nursing in Connecticut in the early 1900s, the simulator was manufactured by New England's Chase Doll Company. Mrs. Chase and her derivative mannequins were commercially produced and used to train nurses until the 1970s (Doyle, 2011a).

Role-play—Role-play has been used in nursing education for many years, especially for developing therapeutic communication skills. Learners are traditionally grouped in dyads or triads to practice and observe case-based scenarios where difficulty in communication might occur. Creating the opportunity to "say" what is inside one's head does not always result in the interaction proceeding as one might imagine. Role-play demonstrations provide participants and observers with "practice" time under minimal pressure, because they are usually done without the context of performing clinical duties. Constructive feedback from peers and expert practitioners is provided in a timely and specific manner to facilitate learning.

Games—Games range from something as simple as a crossword puzzle of medical terms to virtual worlds that simulate a highly sophisticated care environment, such as an emergency department.

Computer-assisted instruction—The use of computer-assisted instruction began in the 1970s. This form of simulation has gained wide adoption, with numerous products now available for health care education and training, including online learning laboratories that facilitate interdisciplinary learning.

Standardized patients—Standardized patients (SPs) involve the use of "patient actors" who, after specialized training, interact with health care professionals learning to take histories or perform physical examinations. Widely used in medical schools, the primary limitation of SPs is their inability to replicate actual pathophysiology. The use of SPs is still limited in schools of nursing but, despite the high cost, is gaining popularity at the graduate level. At present, many programs use hybrid simulation, which combines two or more simulation modalities into one education and training activity. An example is using an SP for interviewing and examination, followed by use of a partial task trainer or patient simulator for further assessment and intervention (Doyle, 2011a).

Virtual reality and haptic-based systems—Virtual reality simulation uses computers to replicate actual procedures, such as surgery or insertion of an IV. Given limitations in the current state of technology and the cost of producing a single module—one procedure—

the promise of virtual reality for use in health care training has not yet materialized. One example of virtual reality, used since the mid-1990s, is computerized trainers that use haptic, tactile simulation to help students learn how to catheterize a vein.

Integrated simulators—Low- through high-fidelity simulators (instructor-driven and model-driven) (Nehring, 2010, p. 8).

High-Fidelity Patient Simulation

High-fidelity patient simulation (HFPS; see Figure 8.1) has been used in the last 10–15 years in schools of medicine, schools of nursing, emergency medical technician training, and training for military health care personnel. HFPS is increasingly being used in hospitals to assess, develop, and assure competence and confidence; for quality improvement activities; and to test system and policy issues.

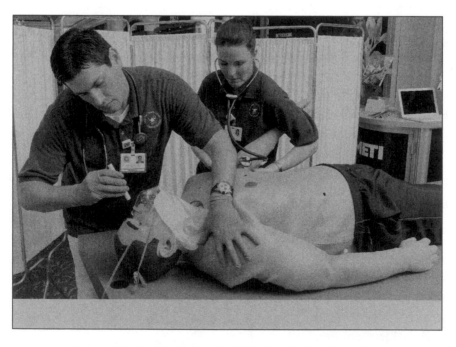

Figure 8.1   Example of a High Fidelity Patient Simulator

Developing Clinical Competence and Confidence

Numerous reasons for adopting HFPS exist, many a direct result of a fast-paced, ever-changing health care delivery system. A primary driver for using HFPS to train caregivers, however, is the modality's effectiveness in providing an environment centered around learners that enables learners to learn and practice the skills and clinical reasoning necessary for safe and effective patient care. Deliberate practice within HFPS is key to developing clinical competence (McGaghie, Issenberg, Petrusa, & Scalese, 2006). In "real" clinical environments, learners are often not given the opportunity to perform—much less practice—the various technical skills required for effective nursing care. This might be because a specific aspect of care that needs to be addressed on a particular day of clinical is not represented in that day's patient population. Or perhaps preceptors are unable to devote attention to monitoring development of a particular skill because of competing demands for their attention from the patient care environment. With HFPS, those hurdles can be bypassed by intertwining the technical skills associated with effective nursing care with challenging opportunities to develop clinical reasoning (Doyle, 2011b). It is well established that "practice makes perfect" (McGaghie et al., 2006). HFPS allows learners to make, detect, and correct patient care errors in a safe, controlled environment without harming patients.

Freed from the inhibiting fear of harming a patient, the learner is empowered, regardless of the rightness or wrongness of a decision, to develop critical thinking abilities and implement decisions accordingly. Learners can then see the outcome of their decisions and reflect on why and what they were thinking and how they would do things differently when faced with a similar situation in the future (Doyle, 2011b).

Facilitating Clinical Judgment

Christine Tanner (2006) defines *clinical judgment* as "the interpretation or conclusion about a patient's needs, concerns, or health problems, and/or the decision to take action (or not), use or modify standard approaches, or improvise new ones as deemed appropriate by the patient's response" (p. 204). HFPS provides an enriched setting where decision-making is required within a complex and ambiguous system. The ability to understand the salient aspects of the situation and respond appropriately in an individualized manner is a skill that is honed over time. Expertise is developed over time by having multiple exposures to diverse cases. This experiential knowledge that nurses carry with them influences their current ability to make decisions (Tanner, 2006). HFPS provides an opportunity to standardize the experiential exposure for all participants in an effort to build the knowledge base. It creates an environment where nurses can conduct deliberate practice on low-volume, problem-prone patient cases to improve decision-making in areas that would normally take years to attain.

Developing Situation Awareness and Clinical Reasoning

The ever-changing dynamics of the practice setting mandate that health care practitioners develop a new skill set of flexibility to adapt to the risk, uncertainty, and pace of patient care. Deficiencies in the ability to make effective or efficient use of information for clinical decision-making can negatively impact nurses' ability to maintain safe patient care. The ongoing surveillance of care is perhaps the most important role that the nurse plays in maintaining patient safety. Preparing nurses to excel in this assessment ability is the essence of situation awareness.

Mica Endsley (1997) defines situation awareness as "being aware of what is happening around you and understanding what that information means to you now and in the future" (p. 13). Situation awareness is heavily influenced by goals and is context-specific: changing as the environment changes. Assessment data is collected and continuously prioritized based on the nurse's understanding of the current goals. This prioritization can be negatively impacted by factors such as stress, workload, complexity, and automation. Assessment data and analysis of that data form the basis for a clinician's ability to make decisions.

Clinical reasoning is a term that refers to the nurse's ability to capture patient trends as a situation changes and take into account the specific patient needs and concerns when formulating a response or action plan for intervention (Benner, Sutphen, Leonard, & Day, 2010). Reasoning is usually developed over years of experience, cultivated by unique patient care experiences rather than didactic learning. HFPS can create specific patient care experiences that learners might never be able to experience, such as blood transfusion reaction, and allow for development of reasoning based on a patient care experience.

HFPS allows the conduction of case-based learning under "real-life" pressures of time, consequence, and prioritization. This type of learning supports the improvement of a practitioner's ability to perceive and comprehend data with the fidelity of time and high-stake consequences. HFPS creates opportunities to understand what augments decision-making and what interferes with the ability to make decisions. It is this understanding that allows learners to create patterns of "knowing" or mental models of patient care that will improve the speed of decision-making in the future.

The hierarchy of learning pyramid developed by METI captures the richness of the simulation learning experience that a new practitioner undergoes throughout the precepted experience (see Figure 8.2). Simulation in particular gives learners the ability to practice knowledge application within the context of collaboration and teamwork of patient care. The briefing and debriefing events of a simulated clinical experience add the richness of expert mentoring to provide assistance with time management, prioritization, and problem-solving skills. Patient care safety is enhanced throughout the experience that learners receive as they fluidly transition between the levels to reinforce their knowledge or sharpen clinical skills.

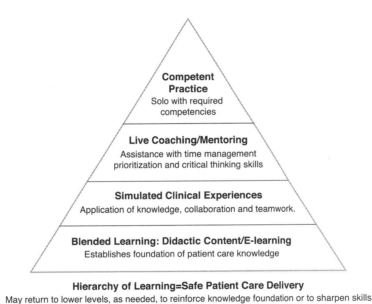

Competent Practice
Solo with required competencies

Live Coaching/Mentoring
Assistance with time management prioritization and critical thinking skills

Simulated Clinical Experiences
Application of knowledge, collaboration and teamwork.

Blended Learning: Didactic Content/E-learning
Establishes foundation of patient care knowledge

Hierarchy of Learning=Safe Patient Care Delivery
May return to lower levels, as needed, to reinforce knowledge foundation or to sharpen skills

Figure 8.2   Hierarchy of Learning Pyramid.
Source: METI, copyright 2010.

Design of High-Fidelity Patient Simulation Experiences

Creating an optimal HFPS learning experience involves goal-oriented learning supported by strong pedagogical principles (Jeffries, 2005). In other words, preceptors and instructors need to know what they are doing and what they expect to attain as an outcome of their teaching. The Jeffries model supports that the HFPS experience should pay particular attention to the maintenance of fidelity while scaffolding learning opportunities through a multiphased approach that minimally includes debriefing (Jeffries, 2005).

The design of the HFPS creates an overlapping richness to the experience, allowing learners to develop their own individual understanding, formulate team goals, and end with reflection on action to create improvements for future patient care.

An HFPS learning event has three key components: foundational knowledge assurance/ briefing, HFPS practice, and debriefing/reflection. Each phase provides the learner with unique experiences for knowledge construction, skill practice, and reflection on action.

Foundational Knowledge Assurance/Briefing

Nursing learning is not a linear application of theory to practice. It is a complex process that requires individualization and modification of knowledge to meet specific clinical situations and to respond to the specific context (Benner, 1984, 1991; Kim, 1999). Individualized care must be balanced with routine tasks in a delicately prioritized manner to maintain patient safety. With HFPS, educators can duplicate this environment for the purpose of creating learning opportunities that enrich the decision-making capacity of the participants.

The briefing stage of simulation practice allows participants to actively create a plan for the individualized care of the patient. Minimally, the environment, roles, goals, and social interactions necessary for a successful nurse-patient interaction should be reviewed and defined during this phase. Prebriefing has been used extensively in aviation practice to mediate the potential for deterioration of situation awareness in situations involving high-cognitive demands, ambiguity, and time pressure (Orasanu & Fischer, 1997). The facilitator guides the process, providing expertise in the form of rich description of theory and experience to highlight the pertinent aspects of clinical practice related to standards and culture. The amount and duration of this guidance are dependent upon the practice level of the participant (i.e., novice, advanced beginner, expert). It can involve the introduction and/ or reinforcement of standards of practice, policies, and procedures that are augmented by the HFPS scenario.

Briefing provides learners an opportunity to defend and explain their understanding of care priorities as part of a larger group and helps them move beyond memorized facts toward an evolving understanding of care that is inclusive and collaborative. Briefing provides the team with the opportunity to formulate specific, consensus-driven goals. The collaborative understanding that is developed during this stage provides the basis for competent action during the HFPS practice.

HFPS Simulation Practice

Jeffries & Rizzolo (2006) found that learning using HFPS promotes a heightened sense of reality, provides opportunity for problem solving, and allows for active and diverse ways of learning. The results of their study also showed that the outcomes of learner satisfaction and self-confidence are rated higher when HFPS is used to conduct clinical training.

Simulation provides learners with an opportunity to apply a collaborative plan along with their individual knowledge in a dynamically changing environment. The simulator's responses are subject to the learner's interventions, and the interventions are dependent upon the patient's response within the environment. It is this reciprocal relationship and evolving awareness that creates the opportunity to practice clinical reasoning during the HFPS practice.

Debriefing/Reflective Practice

Nursing as a profession requires practitioners to continually use their experiences to improve their skills. Reflective practice is one of the tools used by the nursing profession to promote a continual focus on lifelong learning (Kim, 1999; Ruth-Sahd, 2003). According to McDonnell and colleagues (1997), debriefing should promote participant self-assessment along with critical thinking and analysis. The debriefing process should focus on relating practice to standards of care and goals rather than an individual participant's performance (Scherer, Bruce, Graves, & Erdley, 2003). All these studies support the importance of a debriefing process post simulation performance.

The design of the debriefing process is essential to the development of important situation awareness and reflection-on-action skills. Reflection includes three key steps: (a) self-awareness; (b) critical analysis of action, knowledge, and feelings; and (c) development of a new perspective resulting in a behavior change (Atkins & Murphy, 1993; Ruth-Sahd, 2003). Kim (1999) describes the reflection process as critical reflective inquiry and notes three ultimate goals: (a) to understand practice in the context of a practitioner, (b) to correct and improve practice, and (c) to generate models of "good" practice.

Debriefing should highlight the specific cues, patterns, inferences, and information that were required to make clinical decisions during the HFPS practice. Understanding how to deconstruct complex tasks into basic elements is difficult for both novices and experts, but for different reasons. Novices have difficulty because their experiential base is limited and might not allow them to understand the subtlety of the evolving clinical situation (Benner, 1984). Experts, on the other hand, have difficulty with deconstruction because their intuition-based practice has embedded the fine details deeply within their long-term memory, creating an instantaneous pattern recognition that evokes action without thinking. Debriefing that includes reviewing the recorded simulation performance provides for a richer opportunity to highlight decision-making in terms of cues, patterns, and inferences that are part of developing situation awareness. The debriefing phase also provides deliberate practice of reflection-on-action skills and team communication skills. Both are essential to the delivery of safe patient care within a complex, team-oriented system.

Implications of Using High-Fidelity Patient Simulation for Preceptors, Educators, and Managers

Using high fidelity patient simulation has many implications for preceptors, educators, and managers. This section includes a review of many of those implications.

Preceptors

Traditional nursing learning utilizes an apprenticeship model characterized by a novice becoming acculturated to the community of practice with the guidance of an experienced expert (Benner, 1984; Lave & Wenger, 1991). This results in a progressive engagement with the clinical practice that allows the novice to move from "lurking and observing" around the periphery to becoming an active member of the community (Lave & Wenger, 1991). During this transition, learners transform their identities through the practice of nursing and gain knowledge and expertise by having experiences with the context, tools, and social practices they have encountered (Benner, 1984; Lave & Wenger, 1991). The learning is part of the richness of practice and is developed and changed by the interaction itself. Expertise traditionally takes place over years as learners gain experience based on naturally occurring interactions with patients, disease processes, and situations within the hospital environment. HFPS provides standardized learning opportunities that can shorten the learning curve and standardize the learning outcomes of health care workers.

Ethics—Because learning in nursing is a socially embedded and shaped practice, it follows that the knowledge, skills, and tools used are vetted by the professional culture and specialty-specific sub-cultures within the practice (Benner, 2000; Benner, Tanner, & Chesla, 1997; Kim, 1999). The preceptor plays a key role in the socialization of preceptees with respect to ethics and knowledge development as they transition from a new graduate role into professional practice or into specialty practice as an experienced nurse. "Common meanings" of what is "good" and "right" come from this social culture and become part of the nurse's guiding value system that influences clinical decision-making (Benner, 2000; Benner et al., 1997; Kim, 1999).

Caring and clinical knowledge are embedded in the pooled expertise and power of multiple perspectives modeled by preceptors. The active modeling process contributes to the shared vision of excellence and strengthens the relationships to establish trust and a sense of possibility between the learner and his/her preceptor (Benner, 2000). Preceptors create inclusion through their transformational stories of excellent patient care and thus promote the cultural norms and values during these interactions.

HFPS creates an opportunity in which ethical decision-making can be practiced and explored within a safe environment. The choice of simulated learning experiences can augment moral development by providing realistic portrayals of end-of-life conflicts, pain management dilemmas, and crisis management instances. The preceptor needs to match the clinical learning experiences with those that are taking place during HFPS to create a realism that helps transition the learning out of the simulation and to the bedside. Exemplars and storytelling are common ways that preceptors assist their preceptees in making the connections between classroom learning and clinical practice. These stories not only solidify that the simulated learning experiences could "really happen," but they also pass along the cultural and ethical norms of the preceptor's practice and that of the nursing unit.

Creating and maintaining a culture of patient safety require diligence for continual improvement. HFPS used during onboarding and competency development can often identify system deficits that require attention. Preceptors need to create dialogue around the gaps that are discovered to improve clinical practice. Preceptees have the opportunity to reshape cultural practice and should be encouraged to discuss their observations regarding gaps among policy, procedure, and clinical practice. This type of inquiry can prove to be challenging to preceptors, but should be viewed as an opportunity to improve practice. Preceptors should take these opportunities to coach to enhance understanding for situations that might necessitate deviation from the norms. By taking time to point out a patient's unique history or by highlighting the ambiguity within a specific patient care situation, preceptors can augment the development of situation awareness outside of the simulation lab.

Knowledge development—Novice practitioners have deficiencies in their ability to make effective or efficient use of available information, to estimate risk and uncertainty, and to select a course of action (del Bueno, 2005; Shanteau, Grier, Johnson, & Berner, 1991). As they gain expertise, nurses change the way they think and apply skills in three distinctive ways: (a) reliance on concrete, experience-based paradigms instead of abstract principles; (b) ability to view the event holistically, instead of as distinct, concrete parts; and (c) movement into care as an active practitioner instead of a detached observer (Benner, 1984). Experts spend the majority of their decision-making time in the assessment and classification of a situation rather than performing lengthy analysis of potential courses of action (Endsley, Bolte, & Jones, 2003). Working off "their gut reaction" or "intuition," experts can adapt quickly to the environment and/or a patient-specific situations.

A common frustration of preceptees is that the preceptor doesn't explain his or her decision-making process. The debriefing phase of HFPS focuses on teaching learners how to deconstruct their clinical performance to understand the cues, patterns, and decisions that were used to take action. Making connections between assessment data and the rationale for decision-making is an important step toward formulating the mental models of experts. Preceptors need to continue this practice of deconstruction in the clinical setting. Verbalization protocols, or "talk out loud" procedures, can help learners understand the subtle cues, patterns, and priorities that the preceptor is attending to prior to making decisions. It is this level of knowledge detail that is essential to the development of clinical expertise over time.

Educators

The influence of facilitators/educators on the simulation learning experience is important. As expert practitioners, they facilitate learning during the briefing and debriefing phases to encourage active participation by all members, using their expertise to gently guide the learning process.

Fidelity—The importance of fidelity has been discussed in detail as an essential component of HFPS learning. The fidelity must represent believable and recognizable occurrences so that participants can be expected to react as they would in the real environment (Wickens, 2000). Environmental and equipment fidelity are usually easily identified and accomplished. After each simulation, educators need to reflect on what could be done to make the experience more realistic. The equipment and supplies used at the bedside must be continually updated in the simulation setting to maintain the realism necessary to allow for clinical immersion for the participants. Psychological fidelity develops over time as the educator develops expertise with the tool of HFPS. Educators' personal clinical experiences come into play here by providing subtle nuances to the responses of the patient or creating family dynamics that are not in the original scripting of the scenario. These embellishments usually do not occur until educators are comfortable in the role of facilitator and with the mechanics of running or working with the simulator. Time and practice using HFPS create comfort and expertise; the important piece is starting somewhere and having a continuous improvement focus.

Facilitation—If one of the goals of HFPS is to create learners who can "think on their feet" and make decisions under time pressure, then the role of the facilitator is to create an environment that promotes construction of knowledge and a propensity toward action.

Facilitation requires a focus on providing timely and specific feedback, encouraging reflective practice, and using a Socratic process to allow for learner construction of knowledge. This is very different from creating a lecture that highlights all the pertinent information that learners need to know about the care of a specific type of patient. Educators need to have a clear understanding of the global goals of the HFPS practice and keep the focus of the learning experience on attainment of those goals.

Facilitation takes place in all three stages of the HFPS practice. The key is to remember to be learner-centered. This means that educators create opportunities for learners to explore and construct their knowledge. During the briefing and debriefing phases, these efforts are focused on drawing out the individual knowledge of each learner while facilitating the distributed knowledge and consensus building of the group toward shared goals and/or shared understandings. During the simulation performance phase, it means letting the team care for the patient with minimal intervention from the expert teacher. This observation piece is often the hardest for educators to do. HFPS is not about doing things perfectly, and it is more than just performing tasks according to procedure. HFPS learning is messy and often goes in a direction that is not expected or intended because it is based on the learners' choices, perhaps what educators fear most. Educators need to understand that their role as observers is to guide the learning toward the global goals while being able to capture some of the unique learning experiences from each group.

Lastly, facilitation is about maintaining the safety of the learning event. If HFPS is going to work as a medium for learning, then failure has to be allowed and accepted as an opportunity for growth. The facilitator creates the environment that supports risk taking and exploration for improvement. This should minimally involve contracting for confidentiality prior to engaging in HFPS teaching.

Adaptation—Too often in health care, the end goal of training is seen as a static set of core competencies. The tool of HFPS suggests that there should be a re-evaluation of that thought process to look at the ability to maintain a flexible and adaptive approach to learning as the end objective of teaching. Minimally, health care settings should begin to add adaptation as a desired core competency. This would require that preceptors, facilitators, and educators adopt the same practice of adaptation within teaching practice to support and role model these important behaviors. HFPS provides participants with an ability to see how multiple interventions based on sound theoretical knowledge can result in the same outcome. It is this expertise that is so necessary for today's practice environment.

Managers

Creating and maintaining a process for educating preceptees are core responsibilities of managers. Onboarding and competency training with HFPS is a resource-intense process. It depends upon having structured time in the simulation lab valued in the same way that clinical experience time is valued. It also requires a commitment to stable preceptor resources. Using preceptors who understand what core competencies are being highlighted within the HFPS experiences helps create a transfer of learning between the simulation setting and into the clinical setting. Managers who understand the importance of creating schedules that maintain the integrity of the preceptor assignment create better learning experiences for preceptees.

Quality Improvement

Every hospital has a process for evaluation of preceptees. Minimally, it is conducted through informal discussions among educators, preceptors, and managers. Decisions are made about length of onboarding and competency development and readiness to perform job duties based on the answers obtained from these conversations. Retrospective reviews are often conducted after training has occurred with the goal of process improvement for the operational structure of orientation.

Using HFPS as a core methodology for onboarding and ongoing competency validation allows for a more formalized approach to the performance evaluation of the preceptee. Collection of concurrent data about readiness to perform, self-confidence levels, and actual clinical performance provides a more objective assessment of the preceptee's performance. This approach involves a 360-degree review of the preceptee from the educator, preceptor, manager, and learner viewpoints.

This type of evaluation data allows the preceptor, manager, and/or educator to intervene in an ongoing manner to create individualized developmental planning for preceptees who aren't meeting standards. Concurrent data can also be used to customize the length of time required based on concrete data rather than anecdotal discussions. HFPS provides learning experiences throughout the onboarding and competency development training to place preceptees under time and high stakes pressure that might not happen on the unit. This type of experience demonstrates the decision-making capacity of preceptees and creates a richer evaluation of their adaptation and readiness to perform the role of direct care nurse.

New Learners—The Net Generation

The Net Generation, those who were born in the 1980s, has grown up within a world that is rich with technology. They are connected 24/7, to each other and globally, through devices that make communication instantaneous and engaging. Information technology has always been a part of their lives in a way that removes the barriers of time and space and creates opportunities for endless learning. Yet, because technology has become so seamless to their daily existence, they just see it "normal." This can be a challenge to preceptors from older generations who are not digital natives and are not as comfortable with newer technologies.

Tapscott (1998) describes Net Generation members as independent, innovative, inclusive, and open. These learners value the autonomy of an active learning process that allows for innovation and creativity when learning. Working in groups where knowledge can be shared, explored, and recreated while valuing the diversity of multiple viewpoints is a preferred style for the Net Generation. Net Generation learners use tools that promote openness, allow for free expression, and provide immediate results in their search for knowledge. The digital literacy of this group allows for widespread access to devices that help them navigate their learning. Net learners are often observed moving seamlessly from the virtual world to the real world while multitasking from one activity to another or, better yet, performing them simultaneously (Skiba & Barton, 2006). Henry Jenkins (2006, p. 3) defines these characteristics as being part of a participatory culture, "a culture with relatively low barriers to artistic expression and civic engagement, strong support for creating and sharing one's creations, and some type of informal mentorship whereby what is known by the most experienced is passed along to novices. A participatory culture is one in which members believe their contributions matter, and feel some degree of social connection with one another." Clearly, the needs of these new learners mandate a different approach to assimilation into health care culture than has been taken in the past.

Nursing education within academic and health care settings has begun to use new technologies such as E-learning, social networking tools, and simulation to enhance the traditional apprenticeship model of learning, both to improve onboarding and competency development in general and in response to Net Generation learners' needs. This new combination of educational techniques not only transforms the professional practice of novice nurses, but also has an effect on experienced nurses as they travel together through onboarding and competency development.

Future of Instructional Technology/Future Implications of Instructional Technology Use

Technology promises to play an even larger part in the ongoing education of nurses in the future than it does today. The "participatory" nature of our profession's newest participants, coupled with the expansion of social networking technology, promises to present numerous challenges as we engage in the practice of using the technology. It will be important as a profession for nursing to provide ethical mentorship of the process. Knowledge building and knowledge sharing are two arenas that will be affected most by technology in the near future.

Knowledge sharing for future health care workers becomes an ongoing and just-in-time process. Using technology to create learning management systems needs to become the norm. Policies and procedures will become living documents in these learning management systems in a way that health care providers have always imagined but never had the tools to create. These learning management system platforms will become spaces where cross-professional groups can come together (in formal and informal teams) to complete tasks and refine processes. Our new generation of health care workers will guide us through this transformation and begin to create the ability for a responsive health care system that can proactively meet the needs of our patients. Evidence-based practice that is evolving can be posted, discussed, and piloted in real time using these tools. Many global businesses of today have already begun this transition. It makes sense that health care will follow. Preceptors will be on the forefront of this transformation.

Another avenue of knowledge sharing that is worth noting is the ability to access knowledge seamlessly. The advent of smartphones as the main mobile technology platform creates an opportunity for health care personnel to have the latest evidence-based practice tools at their fingertips. Applications or "apps" enable users to create a personalized palette of tools to enhance care of the patient (i.e., Spanish translation tools and medication calculators). Health care workplaces and personnel will grapple with access and privacy issues as this seamless knowledge becomes more mainstream in the future.

Because creative expression, circulation of information, and social affiliation are such prominent parts of the Net Generation's daily lives, preceptors need to provide these new professionals with an ethical mentorship regarding use of patient care information. Tweets, texts, blogs, and Facebook postings of daily activities are normal for the Net Generation and present a potential danger for patient and hospital privacy. Preceptors play a strong role in shaping the practice in this area. Preceptors need to understand and help define these emerging practices in terms of the ethical implications that evolve. Posting information, as benign as it might seem, creates an area that needs to be monitored, discussed, and reified within the profession. To guide behavior in these affiliation spaces, preceptors and preceptees must have an ongoing conversation that identifies and solidifies patient advocacy and patient privacy.

Clearly, technology is here to stay. The tools discussed in this chapter highlight only a portion of those that are available in today's world. Preceptors, educators, managers, and learners need to continue to have dialogue regarding how to use technology to facilitate the exchange of information and knowledge between preceptors and preceptees, as well as between diverse communities of learners. The challenge will be to understand and maximize the use of new tools that fit within the culture of health care for the benefit of our patients. Preceptors are and will increasingly be at the cutting edge of technology, learning, and patient care.

References

Atkins, S., & Murphy, K. (1993). Reflection: A review of the literature. *Journal of Advanced Nursing, 18*(8), 1188-1192.

Benner, P. (1984). *From novice to expert: Excellence and power in clinical nursing practice.* Menlo Park, CA: Addison-Wesley.

Benner, P. (1991). The role of experience, narrative, and community in skilled ethical comportment. *Advances in Nursing Science, 14*(2), 1-21.

Benner P. (2000). The roles of embodiment, emotion, and lifeworld for rationality and agency in nursing practice. *Nursing Philosophy, 1,* 5-19.

Benner, P., Sutphen, M., Leonard, V., & Day, L. (2010). *Educating nurses: A call for radical transformation.* San Francisco: Jossey-Bass.

Benner, P., Tanner, C. A., & Chesla, C. A. (1997). The social fabric of nursing knowledge. *American Journal of Nursing, 97*(7), 16BBB-16DDD.

Boulos, M. N., Maramba, I., & Wheeler, S. (2006). Wikis, blogs and podcasts: A new generation of web-based tools for virtual collaborative clinical practice and education. *BMC Medical Education, 6*(41), doi: 10.1186/1472-6920-6-41.

Clark, R. C., & Mayer, R. E. (2007). *e-Learning and the science of instruction: Proven guidelines for consumers and designers of multimedia learning.* (2nd ed.). New York, NY: Pfeiffer.

del Bueno, D. (2005). A crisis in critical thinking. *Nursing Education Perspectives, 26*(5), 278-282.

Doyle, T. J. (2011a). Do the patient no harm: Using simulation to prepare nurses for the real world. *Reflections on Nursing Leadership, 37*(2). Retrieved from http://www.reflectionsonnursingleadership.org/Pages/Vol37_2_Doyle_simulation_Part1.aspx

Doyle, T. J. (2011b). Do the patient no harm: Using simulation to prepare nurses for the real world. *Reflections on Nursing Leadership, 37*(2). Retrieved from http://www.reflectionsonnursingleadership.org/Pages/Vol37_2_Doyle_simulation_Part2.aspx

Endsley, M. R. (1997). The role of situation awareness in naturalistic decision-making. In C. E. Zsambok & G. A. Klein (Eds.), *Naturalistic Decision-making* (pp. 269-284). Mahwah, NJ: Lawrence Erlbaum Associates.

Endsley, M. R., Bolte, B., & Jones, D. G. (2003). Designing for situation awareness: An approach to user-centered design. Boca Raton, FL: CRC Press.

Jeffries, P. R. (2005). A framework for designing, implementing, and evaluating simulations used as teaching strategies in nursing. *Nursing Education Perspectives, 26*(2), 96-103.

Jeffries, P. R., & Rizzolo, M. A. (2006). *NLN/Laerdal project summary report, designing and implementing models for the innovative use of simulation to teach nursing care of ill adults and children: A national, multi-site, multi-method study.* Retrieved from http://www.nln.org/research/laerdalreport.pdf

Jenkins, H. (2006). *Confronting the challenges of participatory culture: Media education for the 21st century.* Chicago, IL: MacArthur Foundation.

Kim, H. S. (1999). Critical reflective inquiry for knowledge development in nursing practice. *Journal of Advanced Nursing, 29*(5), 1205-1212.

Lave, J., & Wenger, E. (1991). *Situated learning: Legitimate peripheral participation.* New York, NY: Cambridge University Press.

McDonnell, L. K., Jobe, K. K., & Dismukes, R. K. (1997). *Facilitating LOS debriefings: A training manual.* Retrieved from http://ntl.bts.gov/lib/000/900/962/Final_Training_TM.pdf

McGaghie, W. C., Issenberg, S. B., Petrusa, E. R., & Scalese, R. J. (2006). Effect of practice on standardized learning outcomes in simulation-based medical education. *Medical Education, 40*(8), 792-797. doi: 10.111/j.1365-2929.2006.02528.x

Nehring, W. M. (2010). History of simulation in nursing. In W. M. Nehring and F. R. Lashley (Eds.), *High-fidelity patient simulation in nursing education* (pp. 3-26). Sudbury, MA: Jones and Bartlett.

Oblinger, D. G., & Oblinger, J. L. (2005). Is it age or IT: First steps toward understanding the net generation. In D. G. Oblinger & J. L. Oblinger (Eds.), *Educating the Net Generation* (pp. 2.1-2.20). EDUCAUSE.

Orasanu, J., & Fischer, U. (1997). Finding decision in natural environments: The view from the cockpit. In C. E. Zsambok & G. Klein (Eds.), *Naturalistic decision-making* (pp. 343-357). Mahwah, NJ: Lawrence Erlbaum Associates.

Ruth-Sahd, L. A. (2003). Reflective practice: A critical analysis of data-based studies and implications for nursing education. *Journal of Nursing Education, 42*(11), 488-497.

Scherer, Y. K., Bruce, S. A., Graves, B. T., & Erdley, W. S. (2003). Acute care nurse practitioner education: Enhancing performance through the use of clinical simulation. *American Association of Critical-Care Nurses Clinical Issues, 14*(3), 331-341.

Shanteau, J., Grier, M., Johnson, J., & Berner, E. (1991). Teaching decision-making skills to student nurses. In J. Baron & R. V. Brown (Eds.), *Teaching decision making to adolescents* (pp. 185-206). Hillsdale, NJ: Lawrence Erlbaum Associates.

Skiba, D., & Barton, A. (2006, May 31). Adapting your teaching to accommodate the net generation of learners. *OJIN: The Online Journal of Issues in Nursing, 11*(2), Manuscript 4. doi: 10.3912/OJIN. Vol22No02Man04.

Tanner, C. A. (2006). Thinking like a nurse: A research-based model of clinical judgment in nursing. *Journal of Nursing Education, 45*(6), 204-211.

Tapscott, D. (1998). *Growing up digital: The rise of the Net Generation.* New York: McGraw-Hill.

Wickens, C. D. (2000). The trade-off of design for routine and unexpected performance: Implications of situation awareness. In M. R. Endsley & D. J. Garland (Eds.), *Situation awareness analysis and measurement* (pp. 211-225). Mahwah, NJ: Lawrence Erlbaum Associates.

Preceptor Development Plan
Effectively Using Instructional Technologies

Review the information on effectively using instructional technologies described in this chapter. What are your strengths? In which areas do you need to increase your knowledge and expertise? What is your plan for expanding your knowledge and expertise? What resources are available? Who can help you?

Name:			
E-Learning			
Strengths	Needs	Plan	Resources
Web-Based Collaboration Tools			
Strengths	Needs	Plan	Resources
Simulation—General			
Strengths	Needs	Plan	Resources
Simulation—High Fidelity Patient Simulation			
Strengths	Needs	Plan	Resources

Note: This form and other resources are available at www.RNPreceptor.com.

"Teaching is the highest form of understanding."
–Aristotle

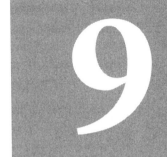

Precepting Specific Learner Populations

Beth Tamplet Ulrich, EdD, RN, FACHE, FAAN

Preceptors work with a number of specific learner populations, each of which has different experiences, knowledge, and needs. This chapter discusses those populations: student nurses on their clinical rotations; new graduate nurses; experienced nurses (changing specialties, returning to practice, learning new roles); internationally educated nurses; and nurses from different generations.

Pre-Licensure Student Nurses

Schools can only teach so much information in didactic classes, skills laboratories, and simulation centers. At some point, the student nurse must experience caring for live patients in health care organizations. To accomplish that, schools of nursing enter into agreements with hospitals and other health care agencies to provide clinical rotations for their students. In most cases, the student rotations are coordinated by a designated person in the nursing department to assure that the number of student rotations does not exceed the capacity of the hospital.

It takes a lot of patience and time to precept student nurses (especially pre-licensure students early in their education), and the role should not be accepted without a lot of thought. I once moderated a panel of nursing faculty, hospital educators and staff, and student representatives in a discussion about clinical rotations. One student was very quiet through most of the discussion, and I

OBJECTIVES

- Understand the needs of specific learner populations

- Individualize precepting based on the needs of specific learner populations

asked her what her thoughts were. She said, "My friends and I just don't understand why we can't be assigned to nurses who like to work with students." The room went dead silent—such a simple request with such big implications. The student went on to describe a recent clinical experience during which, after she handed off the patient, the nurse she was assigned to did not speak to her the rest of the time she was there—certainly not the way we want to bring young nurses into our profession. The student was right—the first criteria for precepting students should be that the preceptor enjoys that role.

The school of nursing, the health care organization, the faculty member, the preceptor, and the student all have responsibilities in a student clinical rotation that should be delineated in written format and shared with all stakeholders. An example of these responsibilities is provided in Table 9.1 by Dr. Anne McNamara, dean of the Grand Canyon University College of Nursing and Health Sciences.

Table 9.1   Grand Canyon University College of Nursing and Health Sciences Guidelines for Preceptor Experience

The College of Nursing agrees to:

- Offer an approved program of study for pre-licensure nursing students that is in accordance with the accepted standards for accreditation.

- Be responsible for planning with the preceptor and agency administration the experiences that will facilitate meeting the learning needs of the student.

- Nursing projects and/or studies made by students in partial fulfillment of the requirements for their degree will always require mutual agreement between the faculty of the College of Nursing and the preceptor.

- Require that students are covered by malpractice insurance.

- Require that students carry health insurance, current CPR validation, and maintain health requirements.

- Require that students write their professional learning objectives for preceptorship experience, final approval of which rests with the designated preceptor and the faculty.

The Agency agrees to:

- Allow students the opportunity to assume a practice role as learning experience within the confines of the clinical setting.

- Allow students to develop their own learning objectives for preceptorship in collaboration with preceptor and faculty within the parameters of the agency.

- Allow students the freedom to independently and/or collaboratively apply the skills of assessing, planning, implementing, and evaluating their own nursing practice.
- Utilize in collaboration with the College the following criteria in selecting student preceptor.

The Preceptor must:

- Have a committed belief in the expanded role of the professional nurse.
- Be bachelor's prepared (BSN) or demonstrate expertise in the field of practice.
- Be willing to serve as preceptor for the necessary time allotment.
- Be willing for the student to pursue individual learning objectives within the parameters of the agency.
- Be willing to assume responsibility for making student assignments for independent practice with careful attention given to the scope of his/her knowledge and skills.
- Supply a written evaluation of student performance (form will be supplied).
- Be licensed to practice nursing in the state of employment.

The Preceptor agrees to:

- Review the preceptorship documents provided by the student and sign the Preceptor Agreement form and the Medication Administration Guidelines form.
- Provide opportunities for the student to pursue individual learning objectives within the parameters of the agency and in accord with the nursing role assumed by the preceptor.
- Allow the student the freedom to independently and/or collaboratively apply the skills of assessing, planning, implementing, and evaluating their own nursing practice.
- Provide opportunities for the student to assume a leadership role as a learning experience within the confines of the practice setting.
- Serve as a resource person, consultant, and supervisor for student's clinical nursing experience.
- Require a written composite copy of student's objectives prior to allowing students to begin clinical experience in the agency.
- Be willing to assume responsibility for making student assignments for independent practice, with careful attention given to the scope of the student's knowledge and skills.
- Provide feedback and evaluation during the experience, including participation in a midterm and a final conference with the clinical faculty, where a rating is made of the accomplishment of each objective. In addition, at the end of the experience, complete a short summary evaluation (form will be supplied).
- Assist faculty in evaluating the preceptorship experience and discuss any needed revision.

Table 9.1	Grand Canyon University College of Nursing and Health Sciences Guidelines for Preceptor Experience (cont.)

The Student agrees to:

- Establish individualized learning objectives for preceptorship experience in collaboration with the clinical faculty and preceptor that are written in measurable behavioral terms. Further, he/she agrees that this activity will be completed as an entry requirement prior to beginning clinical experience for preceptorship.

- Negotiate with preceptor for experiences that will facilitate meeting personal learning objectives and assist in the development of professional competencies.

- Have current health insurance and/or assume the cost of any health care services not covered by insurance.

- Collaborate with preceptor to plan the required contact hours in accordance with the preceptor's schedule.

- Be responsible for obtaining all appropriate signatures on preceptor's letter of agreement.

The Faculty Advisor agrees to:

- Complete all items listed on the Clinical Faculty Checklist throughout the rotation.

- Assist students in refining objectives prior to preceptorship.

- Establish a mechanism for maintaining contact with preceptors during the period of preceptorship when not in the agency. Examples of mechanisms include letters, telephone contact, pager, on-site visits, and conferences.

- Require students to complete self-evaluation, which includes input from preceptor, faculty, and student to determine a final grade.

- Evaluate the student's performance during preceptorship using input obtained from the preceptor and student, as well as specific objectives.

- Grade student papers using specified criteria.

- Communicate weekly with the lead faculty or more often as needed.

- Make site visits as established.

(Used with permission from GCU CNHS)

The school should also provide a preceptor orientation, details of the specific clinical experience (when, what is to be accomplished, etc.), details of the students to be precepted, applicable school policies and procedures, contact information for the faculty, and evaluation forms for the preceptor to evaluate the student and vice versa, as well as for the evaluation of the preceptorship experience in general. The health care agency (hospital, etc.) should have written policies and procedures about nursing student clinical rotations that include any limitations on what students can do during their rotations. For example, the National

Council of State Boards of Nursing (NCSBN), in a 2006 study, found that in 44% of the rotations, students were not allowed to call physicians and in 15%, students did not have the opportunity to supervise the provision of care by others.

Creating a Positive Clinical Learning Environment

After performing an extensive literature review of learning environments in general, Chan (2002, 2003) developed and tested a clinical learning environments inventory. Newton and colleagues (2010) performed a factor analysis on the inventory and identified six factors that account for the dimensions of clinical learning environments that are salient to students.

1. Student-centeredness—The attributes of the clinical teacher in taking time to engage with students individually, to listen, and to offer support to help them achieve their goals.

2. Affordances and engagement—Opportunities afforded to students to actively engage in unit activities and work.

3. Individualization—Students having some control over their clinical experiences and facilitating the achievement of their individual learning needs.

4. Fostering workplace learning—A workplace that fosters learning, with clear, well-planned, and interesting student assignments.

5. Valuing nurses' work—Students recognizing the value of nursing work, making an effort to get their work done and to be regarded favorably.

6. Innovative and adaptive culture—A person-centered approach and a workplace that promotes creative, flexible, and adaptive work practices.

Hartigan-Rogers et al. (2007) studied nursing graduates' perceptions of the effectiveness of their clinical placements and found four themes around the relevancy of the experiences to their future practice.

1. Developing nursing skills and knowledge—There was a high value placed on attaining nursing skills and knowledge, so they wanted clinical placements that provided frequent opportunities to practice all types of skills, including psychomotor, communication, time management, and organizational skills.

2. Experiencing the realities of work life—They wanted realistic patient care situations and workloads.

3. Preparing for future work—They wanted to do the work, not just observe others doing it.

4. Experiencing supportive relationships—They preferred having preceptors and supportive relationships.

A Recruitment Strategy

Precepting nursing students can be a direct investment in the future. Clinical rotations are an excellent way to recruit nursing students for part-time work during school and full-time work when they graduate, and to ascertain whom you want to recruit. New graduates are more likely to seek employment in health care organizations in which they had positive clinical learning experiences. Ulrich (2003), in a longitudinal study of new graduate nurses, found that bonding students to the organization while they were students and letting them know there was a position for them resulted in the students not even looking elsewhere for jobs after graduation.

New Graduate Nurses

Think back to when you graduated from nursing school. How did you feel? The two most frequent words that new graduate nurses use when entering their first job are "excited" and "scared" (Ulrich, 2003). New graduates come into the workplace exhilarated at having accomplished their goals of completing their degrees and passing the NCLEX exam, but anxious about being responsible for patient care.

New graduate nurses who are young in age are also dealing with a number of major life changes—moving away from parents, having to work 40 hours a week or more, balancing work and life. It is helpful to appreciate and remember that becoming a registered nurse is only one of the transitions they are experiencing. As Duchscher (2008, p. 442) says, the first year of work experience "encompasses a complex but relatively predictable array of emotional, intellectual, physical, sociocultural, and developmental issues that in turn feed a progressive and sequential pattern of personal and professional evolution." Kramer (1974) in *Reality Shock* provided the seminal work on the transition of new graduates, work that is still pertinent today. Duchscher (2008) describes the first 12 months of transition as a process of becoming that occurs in three phases (although it is not always a linear process).

1. Doing—Learning, performing, concealing, adjusting, accommodating

2. Being—Searching, examining, doubting, questioning, revealing

3. Knowing—Separating, recovering, exploring, critiquing, accepting

The Practice-Education Gap

In a recent study on educating nurses, Benner and colleagues (2010, p. 4) note that a major finding of their study "is that a significant gap exists between today's nursing practice and the education for that practice, despite some considerable strengths in nursing education." They further state, "Even if nursing and nursing education were to receive an immediate influx of appropriately designated resources to address the shortages, along with appropriate policy changes, it would take many years to yield results" (p. 7).

This same gap has been identified in a number of other studies from a variety of viewpoints. Using the Performance Based Development System (PBDS), del Bueno (2005) reviewed 10 years of data for new nurses and found that 65% to 76% of inexperienced RNs did not meet the expectations for entry-level clinical judgment. Further, the majority had difficulty translating knowledge and theory into practice. A national survey of new graduate nurses conducted in 2004 to 2005 also supported the existence of a gap in new graduate nurses' readiness to practice (Kovner et al., 2007; Pellico, Brewer, & Kovner, 2009). The gap was also identified at the beginning of the Quality and Safety Education for Nurses (QSEN) program (Smith, Cronenwett, & Sherwood, 2007). Finally, in a study for the Advisory Board Company, Berkow and colleagues (2008) surveyed nursing school leaders and hospital nurse executives. When asked for their degree of agreement with the statement "Overall, new graduate nurses are fully prepared to provide safe and effective care in the hospital setting," 89.9% of the nursing school leaders agreed versus only 10.4% of the hospital nurse executives.

Bridging the Gap—Transition to Practice

The evidence continues to mount that all new graduates need a formal transition to practice program to move from the student role to the role of a professional nurse. The NCSBN has developed a Transition to Practice Model that incorporates specialty content, communication, safety, clinical reasoning, prioritizing/organizing, utilization of research, role socialization, and delegating/supervising as well as the QSEN competencies and their accompanying knowledge, skills, and attitudes (NCSBN, 2008).

Benner and colleagues (2010) recommend a 1-year residency program focused on one clinical area of specialization and recommend that the residency include mentoring. Dyess and Sherman (2009) also found that support was needed throughout the first year. Their study was based on data collected from evaluations and focus groups of new graduates who participated in the Novice Nurse Leadership Institute, a community-wide program designed to strengthen the competencies, provide ongoing support, and develop a leadership mind-set of new graduates.

Formal residency programs already in existence substantiate the need for such residencies and the positive outcomes that can be achieved for individual nurses and their organizations (Beyea, Slattery, & von Reyn, 2010; Fink, Krugman, Casey, & Goode, 2008; Ulrich et al., 2010). Outcomes include a dramatic decrease in first-year turnover, accelerated competence and confidence, and increased engagement of new graduate nurses. Keys to the success of these programs are structure, the use of Benner's novice to expert model, an evidence-based curriculum, preceptor-guided clinical experiences, mentoring, recognition, a dedicated residency coordinator/manager, and measurement of outcomes.

It should also be noted that these residency programs occur after the health care organization's orientation program. Orientation is the process of new employee assimilation and socialization into the organization, introducing new employees to the hospital, gathering information, etc. If your organization does not have a formal residency or transition to practice program for new graduates, the components described previously should be incorporated as much as possible when new graduate nurses are hired. You can find information and resources throughout this book and on its accompanying website *(www.RNPreceptor.com)* that can assist you in preparing to precept new graduates.

Precepting New Graduate Nurses

Schumacher (2007) studied how new graduates perceive the caring behaviors of preceptors by analyzing new graduates' daily reflective journal entries and follow-up interviews. Six themes were identified:

1. Advocating—Made sure assignments facilitated good learning experiences; asked questions to understand how the preceptee best learned. Result: The preceptees thought the preceptors were on their side and helped them progress and be successful.

2. Welcoming—Warmly greeted the preceptee; demonstrated open, approachable, and friendly attitudes; encouraged questions and discussions. Result: The preceptees were less anxious and asked questions.

3. Including—Introduced preceptee to other staff; included them in unit activities. Result: Work was a more comfortable and less threatening place.

4. Appropriate preceptor presence—Took the time to gauge preceptees' capabilities and gave them autonomy that was challenging yet appropriate. Result: Preceptees learned and thrived.

5. Making human-to-human connections—Went above and beyond; made deeper human-to-human connections; shared some of the unspoken rules of the nursing culture. Result: Longer term relationships.

6. Genuine feedback—Provided continuous, constructive, nonpunitive, concise, and specifically focused feedback. Result: Preceptees understood the safest and best way to perform patient care.

Managing the Normal Chaos

With new graduates, preceptors need to pay particular attention to helping those graduates manage the normal chaos of a typical nursing unit. They not only have to learn how to take a full patient load, but they also need to learn how to work quickly, how to deal with interruptions, and how to move easily from one task or thought to another. Cornell and colleagues (2010) in a study of nurses on a medical-surgical unit found that the duration of 40% of the nurses' activities was less than 10 seconds, and for about another 25%, the duration was less than 20 seconds. Only 5% of the events lasted longer than 2 minutes. This is a far different pattern than most nursing students experience in school.

Scope of Practice and Autonomy

One of the most basic things for new graduates to understand is their scope of practice—what they are permitted and expected to do within the scope of their licensure as a registered nurse, what they cannot do, and under what conditions. New graduates need to know the scope of practice for individuals who work in other professions and roles (i.e., physician, nurse practitioner, pharmacist, respiratory therapist, certified nursing assistant, licensed vocational/practical nurse). These scopes of practice vary from state to state, so preceptors need to be knowledgeable of the scopes of practice in the state in which the practice is occurring.

New graduates must be precepted with the goal for them to eventually practice to the full scope of their RN license. One aspect of that practice that is often not clear to new graduates is clinical autonomy. Throughout their education, they have always been under the direct or indirect supervision of an instructor or clinical preceptor. The transition to practicing autonomously in many areas is new to them, and they need guidance and support in this transition.

Kramer and colleagues (2006) have analyzed the concept of clinical autonomy and studied nurses' perceptions of autonomy. After an extensive literature review and interviews with nurses, they created the following definition of clinical autonomy: "Autonomy is the freedom to act on what you know in the best interests of the patient—to make independent clinical decisions in the nursing sphere of practice and interdependent decisions in those spheres where nursing overlaps with other disciplines. Autonomy is facilitated through evidence-based practice, being held accountable in a positive, constructive manner, nurse manager support, and it often exceeds standard practice" (p. 480). They further state, "The sine qua non of safe autonomous practice is knowledge and competence" (p. 488). When nurses in the study were asked to identify situations in their unit that commonly required autonomous decision-making by staff nurses, six domains were found:

1. Emergency domain—Saving lives

2. Need to rescue domain—Patient safety and prevention of harm

3. Patient advocacy domain—Advocating for the patient's physical and mental well-being

4. Triage domain—Effective and efficient care

5. End-of-life domain—Maintaining quality of life and promoting a peaceful death

6. Coordinating/integrating domain—Providing holistic care

These domains can be used by preceptors when teaching new graduate nurses when, where, and how they should practice autonomously. In the Kramer et al. (2006) study, it is also relevant to note that levels of expected autonomous practice varied by type of hospital (community or university teaching hospital) and by type of specialty unit (for example, oncology, medical-surgical, intensive care, outpatient). Preceptors, therefore, must be knowledgeable on the norms and expectations of the hospitals and units in which they practice.

Other Considerations With New Graduates

Other things to consider with new graduates include their pre-licensure education and prior work experience in health care, and whether nursing is their first career. Pre-licensure education can be through a diploma program, an associate degree, a bachelor's degree, or an accelerated degree program. The curriculum is different in each. Students also have the opportunity in some schools to do independent study their last year that, depending on the topic, can provide them with more reality-based experience prior to graduation.

Accelerated or second-degree students tend to be very motivated and to be high achievers in school (American Association of Critical-Care Nurses, 2010), but they might also have a more realistic view of what they don't know. Nursing is a very stable and flexible career that pays well compared to many jobs, so it has become attractive as a second career to people who previously chose less stable professions. Though second-career nurses might come to you with more "street smarts" than the young new graduate, remember that they are no less intimidated by their lack of knowledge and expertise. Imagine, as an experienced nurse, if you started a job tomorrow as an elementary school teacher or an accountant. How would you feel about being a total novice again? And when you're a total novice in a hospital, you understand that mistakes can have dire consequences. Prior paid work experience in health care can also be a factor in what preceptees need to learn (or, in some cases, unlearn). Preceptors need to spend sufficient time with preceptees at the beginning of the relationship to understand the experience and knowledge the preceptees received in school, so that their learning needs can be better identified.

Experienced Nurses

When experienced nurses change specialties or roles, they are no longer proficient or expert nurses in their new positions. This includes nurses who want to learn a new specialty or sub-specialty; nurses who move into new roles such as charge nurses, managers, educators, preceptors, and researchers; nurses who become advanced practice nurses; and re-entry nurses. Preceptors are needed for all of these transitions.

Often, health care organizations do not have structured programs for learning new specialties or roles. In some cases, professional nursing organizations have curricula and resources (for example, Association of periOperative Registered Nurses [AORN] and National Nursing Staff Development Organization [NNSDO]) that can be used. Some health care organizations have developed residencies in clinical areas. For example, Massachusetts General Hospital reported the development of an evidence-based nurse residency program in geropalliative care (Lee, Coakley, Dahlin, & Carleton, 2009).

Re-entry nurses have been out of the workforce for a while. How long they've been out and how long they practiced before they left are good indicators for what they will need to learn. If they worked for some time before taking time away, they are probably quite anxious, because they know they're "rusty" and that practices and technologies have changed since they worked. The good news is that they came back because they wanted to, and they generally have a realistic view of what they don't know.

When experienced nurses change specialties or roles, they can feel vulnerable in their new roles until they acquire the new knowledge and expertise to advance back to the proficient and expert stage. Often, the new role can build on prior knowledge, but not always. As with new graduate nurses, the preceptor needs to understand what outcomes are expected from the preceptorship and what the preceptee's prior knowledge and expertise are.

Experienced nurses who are new hires to the organization generally have experience in the area they are hired into. Patient safety requires that the hiring organization be sure that nurses are competent in clinical practice, regardless of the years of experience. As the preceptor for these nurses, you will often be the person to make that assessment and to assure that any deficits are corrected. In addition, every hospital does things a little differently. Nurses might have been experts in their previous role in knowing the policies and procedures of that organization and in knowing the physician practice patterns, but these things will have to be learned in the new organization.

Lucile Packard Children's Hospital at Stanford recently reported on an innovative concept that it implemented to fill the gap between general nursing orientation and unit orientation (Hargreaves, Nichols, Shanks, & Halamak, 2010). Authors of the report identified that preceptors, despite being responsible for documentation of the knowledge and skills of newly hired nurses and their education when needed, were rarely given specific information about the nurses' prior performance in general orientation, which includes didactic information reinforced with simulation and debriefing. Applying the same concepts used with patient handoffs, they created a handoff report card. It includes information from new hire nurses on their prior jobs and self-assessments of their level of expertise, an instructor assessment, and documentation of competency validation. The report card, which is used to document strengths and areas needing improvement, is discussed with each orientee on the last day of orientation and distributed to the orientee's manager and preceptor. In this way, the unit orientation can be customized to build on the findings during general orientation to result in more rapid skill and knowledge acquisition. This is an excellent example of assuring that preceptors have the information they need to assure an effective and efficient preceptorship.

Internationally Educated Nurses

The number of internationally educated nurses practicing in the United States is increasing. In 2007, Buerhaus and colleagues found that employment of internationally born nurses accounted for one-third of the total growth of RN employment in the U.S. labor market in the previous 4 years.

Practice gaps have been identified between internationally educated nurses and nurses educated in the United States in areas such as performance of assessments, pain management, administration of medications, and use of technology (Edwards & Davis, 2006; Ryan, 2003). Gerrish and Griffith (2004) also note that the adjustment to differences in professional practice might be an issue. Sherman and Eggenberger (2008) report that the impact of cultural differences (such as nurse autonomy and accountability) has been an area of concern identified by nurse leaders, and that internationally educated nurses note that collaboration between nurses and physicians is different in different cultures. Adeniran et al. (2008) found that the transition of internationally educated nurses is not difficult because of a lack of knowledge or clinical skills, but because of sociocultural differences, language subtleties, and unfamiliar surroundings. As a result, internationally educated nurses might require an extended preceptorship. Preceptors need to address those issues delineated previously in addition to the standard preceptorship content.

Nurses From Different Generations

It's far different to precept a 20-year-old than a 40-year-old. They were brought up in very different environments and can have very different outlooks on the world in general, and nursing and health care in particular. Though we never want to generalize too much, it is informative to understand the trends within each generation.

According to Hicks and Hicks (1999), values are the key defining variable of each generation. They note, "The values we develop in our youth are the foundation for what we believe as adults" (p. 4). This values development applies not only to children, but also to joining a profession (Ulrich, 2001). Massey (1979) defined three stages of value development: imprinting (observation), modeling (finding heroes—good or bad), and socialization (by peers or significant others). As a preceptor, you might contribute to the modeling stage of values development for student nurses, who will model themselves on nurses they observe, and to the socialization stage for new graduates and experienced nurses moving into new specialties or roles. Zemke and colleagues (2000) also note that the work environment when individuals of a generation look for their first job contributes to the long-term values and character of their generation.

Generations are usually grouped in time periods. Baby Boomers were born from about 1946–1964, Generation X from 1964–1980, and Generation Y/Millennials/Net Generation from 1980–2000.

Baby Boomers were born into nuclear families in a healthy, growing economy with high employment. They were doted on by their parents and encouraged to think independently and express themselves. Defining events in their generation included the Vietnam War, the 1960s drug culture, and the civil rights movement. They were a very large generation in sheer numbers and have heavily influenced all aspects of the culture since their birth.

Generation X, on the other hand, grew up in a time of employment uncertainty, were often "latch-key" kids, and lived in a time when the divorce rate skyrocketed. They learned self-sufficiency and flexibility early in life. They grew up using television as a window on the world and learning from *Sesame Street* and the Learning Channel. Defining events for Generation X included the birth of MTV in 1981, the AIDS epidemic, and the Challenger accident. Birth control, divorce, and the economy together resulted in Generation X being a much smaller generation in number than the Baby Boomers.

Conversely, the Millennial Generation is as large or larger than the Baby Boomer generation. Like Baby Boomers, they were born into a good economy, but were more likely than previous generations to be born to single mothers. They are the most diverse generation and are very technoliterate. They do not remember a time in their lives without computers and the Internet. As a result, members of the Millennial Generation expect to be constantly learning, and indications are that they process information in more of a mosaic (multitasking) pattern. Defining events of the Millennial Generation include Columbine, the Gulf Wars, and September 11, 2001.

As noted previously, each generation develops values based on its environment (Zemke et al., 2000).

- Baby Boomers—Optimism, personal growth, personal gratification, team play

- Generation X—Diversity, balance, technoliteracy, self-reliance

- Millennial Generation—Diversity, optimism, civic duty, achievement

Each generation also brings certain strengths to the workplace (Zemke et al., 2000).

- Baby Boomers—Driven, team players, service-oriented, relationship-oriented

- Generation X—Good with change, multitaskers, technoliterate, not intimidated by authority, self-reliant, creative

- Millennial Generation—Optimistic, want to help others, multitaskers, technoliterate, outcome-driven, like to learn

Learning Styles and Preferences

Putting all of the generational experiences and characteristics together, it is easy to understand that people from different generations often have different learning styles and preferences. Johnson and Romanello (2005) have described some of them:

- Baby Boomers—Enjoy contact with the teacher, used to learning in a didactic format, learn best when their experience can be connected to the subject matter, want to learn in a caring environment, like positive feedback.

- Generation X—Learn quickly and efficiently, want to learn things that benefit them and their careers, like to learn on their terms, value flexibility, like to see a connection between what they need to learn and how they will use it in their careers.

- Millennial Generation—Like working in groups, like using technology whenever possible, enjoy experiential activities, have little to no tolerance for delays and wasted time, like immediate feedback.

By considering these styles and preferences, preceptors can enhance the learning of members of each generation.

Precepting and Working With Each Generation

Members of each generation bring strengths and preferences to learning situations and to work. Knowing the origin of these strengths and preferences contributes to understanding the members of each generation. As a preceptor, this knowledge can help you individualize preceptees' experiences. As a colleague, this knowledge can help you value what each person can contribute to the team and create an awareness of what you can learn from people in each generation.

Conclusion

Preceptors are called upon to work with many different individuals in many different situations. By having knowledge of specific learner populations, preceptors can be better prepared to meet the needs of all learners.

References

Adeniran, R. K., Rich, V. L., Gonzalez, E., Peterson, C., Jost, S., & Gabriel, M. (2008). Transitioning internationally educated nurses for success: A model program. *The Online Journal of Issues in Nursing, 13*(2), Manuscript 3.

American Association of Colleges of Nursing (AACN). (2010). *Accelerated programs: The fast-track to careers in nursing.* Washington, DC: Author. Retrieved from http://www.aacn.nche.edu/Publications/issues/Aug02.htm

Benner, P., Sutphen, M., Leonard, V., & Day, L. (2010). *Educating nurses: A call for radical transformation.* San Francisco, CA: Jossey-Bass.

Berkow, S., Virkstis, K., Stewart, J., & Conway, L. (2008). Assessing new graduate nurse performance. *Journal of Nursing Administration, 38*(11), 468-474.

Beyea, S. C., Slattery, M. J., & von Reyn, L. J. (2010). Outcomes of a simulation-based residency program. *Clinical Simulation in Nursing, 6*(5), 169-175.

Buerhaus, P., Auerbach, D., & Staiger, D. (2007). Recent trends in the registered nurse labor market in the United States: Short-run swings on top of long-term trends. *Nursing Economic$, 25*(2), 59-66.

Chan, D. (2002). Development of the clinical learning environment inventory: Using the theoretical framework of learning environment studies to assess nursing students' perceptions of the hospital as a learning environment. *Journal of Nursing Education, 41*(2), 69-75.

Chan, D. (2003). Validation of the clinical learning environment inventory. *Western Journal of Nursing Research, 25*(5), 519-532.

Cornell, P., Herrin-Griffith, D., Keim, C., Petschonek, S., Sanders, A. M., D'Mello, S., . . . Shepherd, G. Transforming nursing workflow, part 1: The chaotic nature of nursing activities. *Journal of Nursing Administration, 40*(9), 366-373.

del Bueno, D. J. (2005). Why can't new registered nurse graduates think like nurses? *Nursing Education Perspectives, 26*(5), 278-282.

Duchscher, J.B. (2008) A process of becoming: The stages of new nursing graduate professional role transition. *The Journal of Continuing Education in Nursing, 39*(10), 441-450.

Dyess, S. M., & Sherman, R. O. (2009). The first year of practice: New graduate nurses' transition and learning needs. *The Journal of Continuing Education in Nursing, 40*(9), 403-410.

Edwards, P. A., & Davis, C. R. (2006). Internationally educated nurses' perceptions of their clinical competence. *The Journal of Continuing Education in Nursing, 37*(6), 265-269.

Fink, R., Krugman, M., Casey, K., & Goode, C. (2008). The graduate nurse experience: Qualitative residency outcomes. *Journal of Nursing Administration, 38*(7-8), 457-469.

Gerrish, K., & Griffith, V. (2004). Integration of overseas registered nurses: Evaluation of an adaptation program. *Journal of Advanced Nursing, 45*(6), 579-587.

Hargreaves, L., Nichols, A., Shanks, S., & Halamak, L. P. (2010). A handoff report card for general nursing orientation. *Journal of Nursing Administration, 40*(10), 424-431

Hartigan-Rogers, J. A., Cobbett, S. L., Amirault, M. A., & Muise-Davis, M. E. (2007). Nursing graduates' perceptions of their undergraduate clinical placements. *International Journal of Nursing Education Scholarship, 4*(1), 1-12.

Hicks, R., & Hicks, K. (1999). *Boomers, Xers, and other strangers: Understanding the generational differences that divide us.* Wheaton, IL: Tyndale.

Johnson, S. A., & Romanello, M. L. (2005). Generational diversity: Teaching and learning approaches. *Nurse Educator, 30*(5), 212-216.

Kovner, C. T., Brewer, C. S., Fairchild, S., Poornima, S., Kim, H., & Djukic, M. (2007). Newly licensed RNs' characteristics, work attitudes, and intentions to work. *American Journal of Nursing, 107*(9), 58-70.

Kramer, M. (1974). *Reality shock: Why nurses leave nursing.* St. Louis, MO: C.V. Mosby Co.

Kramer, M., Maguire, P., & Schmalenberg, C. E. (2006). Excellence through evidence: The what, when, and where of clinical autonomy. *Journal of Nursing Administration, 36*(10), 479-491.

Lee., S. M., Coakley, E. E., Dahlin, C., & Carleton, P. F. (2009). An evidence-based nurse residency program in geropalliative care. *The Journal of Continuing Education in Nursing, 40*(12), 536-542.

Massey, M. (1979). *The people puzzle: Understanding yourself and others.* Reston, VA: Reston Publishing.

National Council of State Boards of Nursing (NCSBN). (2006). *A national survey on elements of nursing education.* Chicago, IL: Author.

National Council of State Boards of Nursing (NCSBN). (2008). *Toward an evidence-based regulatory model for transitioning new nurses to practice.* Chicago, IL: Author. Retrieved from https://www.ncsbn.org/Pages_from_Leader-to-Leader_FALL08.pdf

Newton, J. M., Jolly, B. C., Ockerby, C. M., & Cross, W. M. (2010). Clinical learning environment inventory: Factor analysis. *Journal of Advanced Nursing, 66*(6), 1371-1381.

Pellico, L. H., Brewer, C. S., & Kovner, C. T. (2009). What newly licensed registered nurses have to say about their first experiences. *Nursing Outlook, 57*(4), 194-203.

Ryan, M. (2003). A buddy program for international nurses. *Journal of Nursing Administration, 33*(6), 350-352.

Schumacher, D. L. (2007). Caring behaviors of preceptors as perceived by new nursing graduate orientees. *Journal for Nurses in Staff Development, 23*(4), 186-192.

Sherman, R. O., & Eggenberger, T. (2008). Transitioning internationally recruited nurses into clinical settings. *The Journal of Continuing Education in Nursing, 39*(12), 535-544.

Smith, E.L., Cronenwett, L. & Sherwood, G. (2007). Current assessments of quality and safety education in nursing. *Nursing Outlook, 55*(3). 132-137.

Ulrich, B.T. (2001). Successfully managing multigenerational work forces. *Seminars for Nurse Managers, 9*(3), 147-153.

Ulrich, B. (2003). Successful strategies for new graduates. *Nurse Leader, 1*(6), 28-30.

Ulrich, B., Krozek, C., Early, S., Ashlock, C. H., Africa, L. M., & Carman, M. L. (2010). Improving retention, confidence, and competence of new graduate nurses: Results from a 10-year longitudinal database. *Nursing Economic$, 28*(6), 363-376.

Zemke, R., Raines, C., & Filipczak, B. (2000). *Generations at work: Managing the clash of veterans, boomers, Xers, and nexters in your workplace.* New York, NY: AMACON.

| Preceptor Development Plan |
| Working with Specific Learner Populations |

Review the information on working with specific learner populations described in this chapter. What are your strengths? In which areas do you need to increase your knowledge and expertise? What is your plan for expanding your knowledge and expertise? What resources are available? Who can help you?

Name:			
Pre-Licensure Student Nurses			
Strengths	Needs	Plan	Resources
New Graduate Nurses			
Strengths	Needs	Plan	Resources
Experienced Nurses			
Strengths	Needs	Plan	Resources
Internationally Educated Nurses			
Strengths	Needs	Plan	Resources
Nurses From Different Generations			
Strengths	Needs	Plan	Resources

Note: This form and other resources are available at www.RNPreceptor.com.

"It's better to light the candle than to curse the darkness."

–Eleanor Roosevelt

Assessing and Addressing Preceptee Behavior and Motivation

Cindy Lefton, PhD, RN

On the drive home, you start analyzing your shift and rehashing the events one by one. Although you can't put your finger on why, a feeling in your gut tells you that your preceptee is struggling. You are not quite sure if this struggle is related to clinical competency issues, connecting with patients, and/or challenges collaborating with other team members. Regardless of the source, the signs and symptoms of a needed attitude or behavioral adjustment can vary. The key here is to "light the candle" by acknowledging your gut feeling and devising a strategy that objectively and constructively addresses the preceptee's issues in a manner that influences behavior change.

Focusing on observable change, this chapter provides you with tools aimed at helping preceptees gain insight regarding how their behavior impacts care delivery, patients, and teammates and identifies strategies you can use to influence their behavior.

Every day, you are surrounded and bombarded by attempts to change your attitudes and behaviors. Billboards, commercials, and advertisements on the homepage of your browser are all attempts to influence your attitude and shift your behaviors. Even your unit's patient satisfaction scores and clinical indicator data posted in

OBJECTIVES

- Increase the effectiveness of preceptee problem-solving strategies

- Assess preceptee behavioral pattern strengths and developmental opportunities

- Implement evidence-based practices to influence preceptee behaviors

- Utilize the Five Step Format as a framework to provide preceptees with action-oriented feedback regarding how their behavior impacts care delivery, patient interactions, and teammates

the breakroom are subtle attempts to impact behaviors of the team. Regardless of the media format, how you receive this information and your behavioral responses to these messages are based upon research arising from the field of psychology.

In essence, psychology is the science devoted to understanding human behavior or, simply, the study of why people do what they do. Since the days of Plato and Aristotle (and probably before), men and women have been trying to unravel the causes of human behavior. Many theories describe the hows and whys of human behavior. Regardless of your theoretical beliefs, the various disciplines of psychology agree that human behavior is both complex and fascinating.

In the hospital setting, where the patient continuum ranges from experiencing life to death, nurses encounter a variety of circumstances where human behavior (what we do and how we do it) saves lives and/or leads to worsening of a condition or possibly a patient death. Over the past decade, a wealth of research has been devoted to exploring the link between patient outcomes and human behaviors (Aiken, Clarke, Sloane, Lake, & Cheney, 2008; American Association of Critical-Care Nurses, 2005; Kohn, Corrigan, & Donaldson, 2000). The consensus is clear that both actions and behaviors impact patient survival as well as the health of our work environments.

Now that data supports the impact of behavior on patient safety, outcomes, and work environments, it is even more critical to address early on those preceptees whose attitudes or behaviors need improvement. Attitudes and behaviors are different. Attitudes are what you think. Behaviors are what you do. Although you can't always see someone's attitude, behaviors are 100% observable. Because behavior is observable, behavioral change is easier to measure. Therefore, most of the tools and strategies in this chapter focus on behavioral change; however, a by-product of behavior change can be an impact on one's attitude (Petrocelli, Clarkson, Tormala, & Hendrix, 2010).

Similar to how you would begin patient care, attitudinal/behavioral improvements should begin with an assessment of the situation. The purpose underlying both patient care and behavioral assessment processes is to identify symptoms and search for causality. For example, when you notice that a patient's urine output is decreased, you assess for hypovolemia, and you might look to see if an issue with kidney function exists, etc. When you encounter a person with a negative attitude or problematic behavior, your assessment often involves attributing these occurrences to internal qualities of the person (Gilbert & Malone, 1995; Heider, 1958). There is often a human tendency to assign negative intentions to people when you encounter problematic situations. This well-documented phenomenon, known as the fundamental attribution error (Gilbert & Malone, 1995; Heider, 1958), can be avoided by increasing your awareness of how you approach problems and by using a framework that promotes a more objective assessment of the situation at hand.

Just Culture: A Problem-Solving Framework

The Just Culture framework can help preceptors objectively assess preceptee performance and guide preceptors away from making fundamental attribution errors. Operating on the premise that the majority of errors occur because of system failures as opposed to individual failures, a Just Culture promotes the philosophy that human beings make mistakes and, instead of jumping immediately to assigning blame, we should encourage exploration of the factors related to the error, make improvements based on these findings, strive to create an environment where candor is valued, and reward people for speaking up to identify events, processes, and behaviors that create safety vulnerabilities (GAIN Working Group E, 2004; Marx, 2008). In other words, a Just Culture emphasizes solving the problem, not attributing negativity or blame.

Though a Just Culture might appear "soft" to some, this type of philosophy does not serve as an excuse for error. Instead, a Just Culture helps avoid attributions and blame by redirecting focus to incorporate both the individual and system contributions to the errors. Organizations supporting a Just Culture still hold employees accountable and responsible for their actions, and they still make a clear distinction between acceptable and unacceptable behaviors (GAIN Working Group E, 2004).

Three Types of Errors

A Just Culture perspective recognizes three different types of errors. The first type, *human error,* involves those situations in which a person was "inadvertently doing something other than what they should have been doing" (Marx, 2008, p. 7) and a slip or a lapse occurs. Human error behaviors might occur, for example, when a preceptee who has been taking care of a patient all day is in a hurry. He or she grabs the CBC label from the printer and checks the name against the patient's ID band, but misses that the birth date is different (unbeknownst to the preceptee, a new patient with the same name was admitted to the floor), and then sends the improperly labeled specimen to the lab. The preceptee should have been paying attention to all the identifiers on the label, but was not concentrating on the task at hand and made a slip.

The second type of error, *at-risk behavior,* encompasses choosing actions that increase the risk of a mistake, "and the risk is not recognized or it is mistakenly believed to be justified" (Marx, 2008, p. 7). An example of at-risk behavior would be a preceptee who identifies that the patient is crashing and attempts to treat the patient without seeking guidance from the preceptor. The preceptee does not seek preceptor guidance because she thinks the preceptor is busy (and doesn't want to bother the preceptor), and views this event as an opportunity to demonstrate that she can handle a high-acuity situation. The mistake in this scenario was that the preceptee convinced herself that demonstrating she can handle the situation and not "bothering" the preceptor was the correct action to take. The preceptee thought she was doing the "right thing," but failed to make the connection between getting the preceptor involved and ensuring patient safety.

The third type of error, *reckless behavior,* involves making a conscious effort to disregard a practice, policy, or norm. This type of error also involves taking a considerable unjustified risk (Marx, 2008). An example of reckless behavior would be a preceptee who does not check the drawn-up dosage of insulin with another nurse. Everyone on the unit is busy and the preceptee is confident she knows how to properly administer medication. She administers the insulin and it's the wrong dose. In this scenario, the preceptee made the choice to be reckless by consciously ignoring and disregarding the double-check, which is a patient-safety best practice.

Applying Just Culture

Applying the Just Culture philosophy as a preceptor allows you to examine preceptee disconnects by dissecting behaviors while avoiding attribution errors. For example, ask yourself if the problems with the preceptee seem to be more related to human error versus at-risk behavior or reckless actions. In the example of the mislabeled specimen, does the preceptee acknowledge that when this error occurred she was thinking about tasks she needed to do for other patients? Not focusing on the task at hand, multitasking, and/or interruptions can lay the groundwork for focus to drift, slip, or lapse, which leads to missing, ignoring, and/or brushing over an important detail (Potter et al., 2005). Coaching the preceptee on the importance of focusing on the patient and providing the preceptee with some multitasking strategies might help the preceptee avoid a potential human error. In this scenario, using the Just Culture framework enables the preceptor to focus on the preceptee's behavior (lack of focus) instead of assigning blame or using energy to "attribute" causality (that is, the preceptee doesn't care, is spacey, doesn't like to care for patients with this diagnosis, etc.).

If you identify that the preceptee is engaging in actions associated with at-risk behavior, this is a red flag that the preceptee needs help in "connecting the dots." In other words, the preceptee needs your help in learning and understanding how certain behaviors can negatively impact a situation. As you help the preceptee connect the dots, you might also identify developmental opportunities around critical reasoning. At-risk behavior can, at times, be mistaken as a symptom of disengagement and carelessness when, in reality, it is a by-product of learning new skills and adapting to a new environment. In the scenario in which the preceptee tried to handle the crashing patient alone, identifying at-risk behavior redirects the focus from attributing actions as being "renegade" to devising coaching strategies that convey the message that in high-acuity situations, delivering nursing excellence often involves a team effort. If you emphasize a learning environment, preceptees demonstrating at-risk behavior might benefit from closer observation and additional coaching. Depending on the severity of the situation and/or the individual preceptee's behavioral trends, at-risk actions might warrant corrective action.

Using the Just Culture framework can also help preceptors identify those situations in which reckless behavior is occurring. Because reckless behavior involves a choice that leads to a blatant disregard for practices, this action is often associated with some form of corrective action. If a preceptee has demonstrated reckless actions, avoiding the attribution error is critical. In these situations, the preceptor's role is to focus on the behaviors linked to the mistake or near miss, and getting the unit manager involved is a must. People exhibiting reckless behavior can turn it around, but management needs to be involved with monitoring preceptee behavior and providing the preceptee with ongoing feedback. Reckless behavior errors are associated with an unjustified risk or action; therefore, statements such as "I meant to do X" or "I was trying to accomplish Y" are not part of this equation. Instead, these types of justifications are associated with at-risk behavior.

The goal of integrating the concept of Just Culture into the preceptor toolbox is to help preceptors avoid placing blame and making attribution errors. In addition to helping preceptors avoid attribution errors, problem solving from the Just Culture perspective emphasizes examining external factors (for example, equipment malfunction, lack of policy, and/or a new physician) as potential sources that could have "set the stage" for behavioral issues to occur (for example, a new physician was covering the unit and did not communicate the order correctly, etc.). Utilizing the Just Culture framework provides preceptors with a more "global view" of the problem at hand. This global perspective can help preceptors identify developmental opportunities for preceptees and might even lead to making some significant improvements that positively impact patient care processes throughout the hospital.

Providing Feedback

Though the Just Culture framework is helpful for identifying problems and guiding preceptors toward solutions, it does not provide any information about delivering the message and/or providing feedback. As a preceptor, part of your role involves creating an environment that promotes learning and allows the preceptee to thrive and become a contributing member of the team. The preceptee is responsible for taking these opportunities to hone his or her skills, grow as a nurse, and become a productive member of the team. You can use feedback as a tool to synchronize preceptor and preceptee responsibilities (Lefton & Buzzotta, 2004; Lefton, Buzzotta, & Sherberg, 1980).

Although feedback serves as a powerful tool, the reality is that you can't change another person's behavior. However, you can influence others to change their behaviors (Cialdini, 2007). Your ability to influence others through feedback is one of the most powerful tools you have as a preceptor. Increasing the success rate of your ability to influence through feedback is, in part, related to your behavioral assessment skills. In other words, you want to ensure that you are influencing the right behavioral patterns and addressing those actions that can lead to errors, poor patient interactions, and ineffective teamwork.

The Dimensional Model of Behavior

The Dimensional Model of Behavior is a tool that preceptors can use to influence behaviors by providing a systematic process to identify preceptee behavioral pattern strengths and developmental opportunities. The information preceptors can glean from using the Dimensional Model of Behavior enables them to influence behavior change by providing preceptees with actionable data based on observations of behavioral patterns, not attributions.

The premise underlying the Dimensional Model of Behavior is that observed workplace behaviors can be broken down into two dimensions—accomplishing tasks and relating to others (Lefton & Buzzotta, 2004; Lefton et al., 1980). The task dimension (see Figure 10.1) helps the preceptor assess how the preceptee goes about accomplishing the work associated with his or her job. The type of task does not matter; it can be inserting a Foley catheter or calling the rapid response team. The emphasis is not on the specific job, but rather on how the preceptee accomplishes the work. In other words, does the preceptee approach the work by demonstrating proactive, dominant, direct, and "make things happen" behaviors? For example, when the preceptee senses an angry family member, does he or she proactively try to understand and problem-solve before the situation escalates? Or, does the preceptee deal with the angry family by taking a more reactive, "let things happen," passive (submissive) approach? In this latter situation, a preceptee might sense the family's frustration but avoid dealing with the family's anger until it explodes.

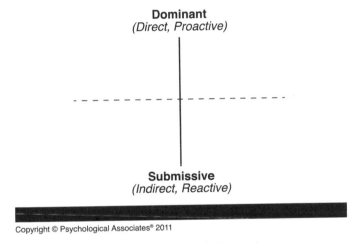

The Task Dimension
Measures how I get things done

Dominant
(Direct, Proactive)

Submissive
(Indirect, Reactive)

Copyright © Psychological Associates® 2011

Figure 10.1   The Task Dimension

The people dimension (see Figure 10.2) assesses how a person conveys warmth and regard toward others. When you assess the people dimension, the focus is on those behaviors you observe as the preceptee interacts with patients and other members of the health care team. In other words, how does the preceptee convey warmth and regard for others? Is she warm, approachable, responsive, and sensitive to the needs of others? Does she give others eye contact? Does she sit down at the bedside and touch the patient? Does she engage in conversations with other staff members? Or, does the preceptee send off a vibe that projects defensiveness, disengagement, disinterest or a noncaring attitude? Does she avoid eye contact with patients and peers, does she respond only to questions that are asked and come across as mechanical? Does she seem to be uncomfortable communicating with other team members?

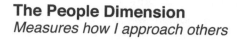

The People Dimension
Measures how I approach others

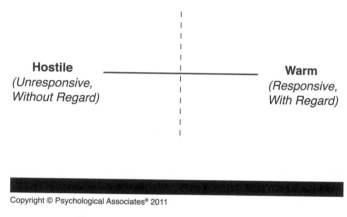

Figure 10.2   The People Dimension

Combining the task and people dimensions of the Dimensional Model of Behavior yields four types (quadrants) of behavior patterns that can describe preceptee behaviors (see Figure 10.3). Individuals tend to exhibit behaviors that reside in one quadrant more than the other three. These are primary behaviors, and individuals rely on these actions more than they do the other behavioral styles. However, depending on the situation, behavior can change, and most everyone from time to time demonstrates actions associated with all four quadrants. For example, when the chief nurse executive calls you into her office, you might exhibit different behaviors than you demonstrate when a peer asks to speak with you. You might observe your preceptee interacting with other preceptees differently than he or she interacts with you. The key point to remember is that everyone is capable of changing behavior, and these changes are influenced by the people you interact with and the situations you encounter. As with any tool such as this, people rarely fit neatly into a box and should always be viewed as individuals. But, the Dimensional Model of Behavior provides the preceptor with a way to systematically look at preceptee behavioral pattern strengths and identify developmental opportunities.

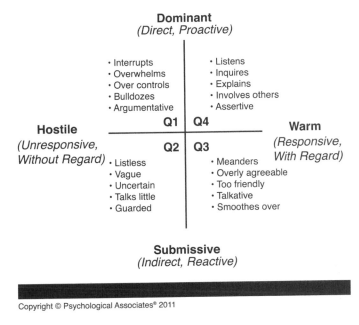

Figure 10.3   Dimensional Model of Behavior

Preceptees who exhibit proactive behaviors and lack of regard for others (quadrant 1–Q1) demonstrate actions that are task-oriented but lack actions that convey sensitivity toward others. Preceptees with primarily proactive and unresponsive behaviors get things done, but they leave a trail of frustrated and often angry people. This occurs because the emphasis on completing tasks overshadows concern and regard for others, and they run over people as they try to get work done. Examples of proactive and lack of regard for others behaviors include interrupting people, arguing, becoming defensive, not being open to the feedback or opinions of others, and a "my way or the highway" attitude. Preceptees exhibiting these behaviors like to "tell and do" and are so focused on getting things done that they often don't realize how insensitive, hostile, and unresponsive they come across to people.

Similar to proactive and lack of regard behaviors, preceptees exhibiting reactive and lack of regard for others behaviors (quadrant 2–Q2) also come across as insensitive, unresponsive, and hostile, but these actions are buffered by their passive and reactive approach to accomplishing tasks. Therefore, these behaviors are often perceived as passive aggressive. Preceptees with a significant amount of reactive and lack of regard for others behaviors are likely to display actions that convey a sense of aloofness; they are often guarded, distant, cool, and noncommittal. Talking to preceptees with a significant amount of these behaviors might feel like "pulling teeth" as you try to get information and input from them. Though their behaviors might convey a sense of disengagement, preceptees with reactive and lack of regard for others behaviors are more comfortable keeping themselves and their emotions close to the vest. They prefer not to "rock the boat," so they tend to follow the rules and stay out of the limelight.

An overdose of warmth, sensitivity, and responsiveness is characteristic of preceptees with reactive and responsive behaviors (quadrant 3–Q3). These overly sensitive behaviors, coupled with a passive approach toward accomplishing the task, yield actions that can be described as too friendly, focusing only on the positive ("optimism on steroids"), and avoiding the negative by glossing over conflict and "sticky issues." Preceptees with predominately reactive and responsive behaviors will eagerly take your feedback and thank you over and over again for the information. However, when it comes to changing their behaviors, if they perceive any conflict associated with altering their actions, they might not follow through.

With an emphasis on both accomplishing the task and valuing others, preceptees with predominately proactive and regard for others behaviors (quadrant 4–Q4) are some of the strongest team members. Preceptees who exhibit these behaviors focus on accomplishing the task but equally value the contributions of others. These proactive and regard for others behaviors are not "soft or fluffy" but, instead, balance the need to accomplish a task with being responsive to teammates. Preceptees with these behaviors will question the preceptor, but do so in a respectful manner that encourages both of you to grow and develop. Behaviors that proactive preceptees with regard for others might demonstrate include providing timely follow-up so you are always in the loop with what's happening with their patients. They are perceived as caring and warm by patients and other staff, and are viewed as engaged, reliable team players. Preceptees with proactive and regard for others behaviors are assertive but not aggressive. They are not afraid to take on a hard assignment and do not hesitate to ask for help. In the event that they get into a situation that is over their heads, they willingly listen to feedback and integrate the preceptor's suggestions into their care delivery.

In summary, the Dimensional Model of Behavior serves the purpose of helping preceptors identify patterns of both effective and ineffective behaviors. Similar to a Just Culture, this model shifts the emphasis away from attribution to observing real-time clinical savvy and interactions among the preceptee, patients, and team members. This kind of observation serves the purpose of providing objective, behavior-based feedback that can enrich the preceptee's experience and gives the preceptee specific examples of behavioral strengths and developmental opportunities. Nurse competencies encompass both clinical expertise and people skills. Identifying the behavioral patterns of your preceptee is the first step in providing meaningful feedback that influences behavioral change. When assessing a preceptee, focus on behaviors you are actually observing. Identify that task orientation first, and then assess the people dimension. When you are assessing your own behavioral patterns, ask yourself, "What are the behaviors I am demonstrating?" This question can help you focus on your actions, not intentions. Finally, always remember the powerful impact your behavior has on the preceptee. Tips for using the Dimensional Model of Behavior are found in Table 10.1.

Table 10.1   Tips for Using the Dimensional Model of Behavior
1. Remember that you are categorizing behavior, not people. A preceptee is not proactive with lack of regard for others (Q1) or reactive with a lack of regard for others (Q2); rather, the preceptee's behavior is in quadrant Q1 or Q2. This is an important concept, because behavior can change.
2. When using the model to assess behavioral patterns, begin by assessing how the preceptee goes about accomplishing the task. Do the preceptee's behaviors appear dominant, proactive, and take a "make things happen" approach? Or, does the preceptee exhibit actions that are more reactive, passive, and take a "let things happen" approach? After you have assessed the preceptee's task behavior, assess behavior in the people dimension—how the preceptee's behaviors convey warmth and regard for others.
3. Observe for behavior changes. As a preceptor, you hold the power in this relationship. This is an important relationship dynamic to understand, because how you use this power can influence preceptee behavior changes. Therefore, you need to increase your awareness regarding how your behaviors impact others. When assessing your own behaviors, don't focus on your intentions (what you want to do) or how you would like to act. Instead, focus on what you are doing and on the actual behaviors you are demonstrating. If you find that you are exhibiting proactive and unresponsive behaviors, your preceptee (as well as other coworkers) might slip into a reactive and lack of regard for others mode or a reactive and regard for others behavioral mode to avoid a confrontation with you. The key is to understand that behavior breeds behavior, and your actions are one of the strongest influencers in your toolbox. As a leader, you owe it to yourself, your preceptee, patients, and team to role-model the behaviors you expect and desire from others.
4. Proactive and responsive actions (Q4) are generally the most effective behaviors, as they balance accomplishing the task with regard for others, and preceptors should find ways of encouraging these actions. Preceptees with proactive and responsive behaviors get things done and do so without leaving a trail of angry and unhappy people.

Motivation

Understanding some basic concepts about motivation (why people do what they do) helps you translate influence into behavior change. In essence, people change behavior based upon their reasons, not necessarily yours (Hall & Lindzey, 1979). Therefore, gaining insight into their reasons or tapping into their motivation can help you influence behavior change and obtain their commitment to a course of action (Perlini & Ward, 2000). Using the model to identify a preceptee's behavioral trends provides you with a window into his or her motivation. In other words, through your behavior you broadcast the reasons for why you do what you do or, rather, why you demonstrate certain behavior patterns, such as those described in the Behavioral Pyramid (see Figure 10.4).

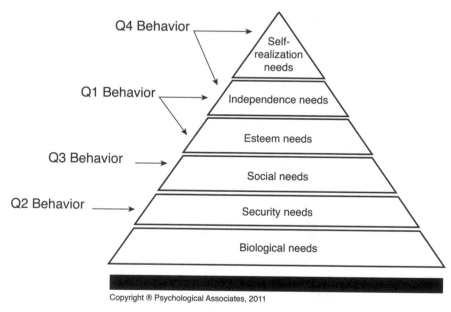

Copyright ® Psychological Associates, 2011

Figure 10.4   The Behavioral Pyramid

Several decades ago, psychologist Abraham Maslow devised a theory to explain how our intangible needs motivate behavior (Hall & Lindzey, 1979). Maslow's theory stated that for individuals to move up the hierarchy of needs, they must satisfy the lower level needs (at the bottom of the pyramid) before they can advance to the next level. Similar to Maslow's model, the Behavioral Pyramid focuses on needs associated with the workplace (Lefton & Buzzotta, 2004; Lefton et al., 1980). For example, workers must first satisfy their biological needs (food, water, etc.) before they can become productive contributors. After these needs have been met, a person can advance to the next level in the hierarchy, security needs (for example, safety, an income, role stability, clarity, and predictability). After these needs have been met, individuals are ready to advance to social needs that center around the desire to be connected with co-workers and create meaningful relationships at work. Upon meeting social needs, individuals can advance to the esteem needs (for example, achievement, recognition for their contributions, and respect from colleagues). After these needs have been met, the individual can progress upward and focus on meeting independence needs, which involve the desire for autonomy and control. Though independence needs are not a part of Maslow's hierarchy, these needs are associated with factors that motivate workplace behaviors (Lefton & Buzzotta, 2004; Lefton et al., 1980). The next level, self-realization, is rarely attained because everyone is always growing. Needs at the self-realization level are associated with obtaining goals that are related to the greater good of the organization and mankind.

Applying the Dimensional Model of Behavior to the Behavioral Pyramid, you can link behaviors to satisfying various needs. Focusing on the reactive and lack of regard behaviors (Q2), a link exists between these actions and the need to establish and maintain security. Preceptees with predominantly reactive and lack of regard for others behaviors are motivated by actions that ensure security, stability, and predictability. These preceptees value policies and procedures because they add a level of predictability and security to the job. From a behavioral change perspective, to influence a preceptee with reactive and lack of regard for others behaviors, link the desired actions to creating stability and security. For example, you notice that your preceptee is exhibiting some reactive and lack of regard for others behaviors. She often eats alone and does not get involved with staff conversations. Approaching the preceptee, you can link the desired behavior change (get more involved with coworkers) by explaining that engaging with staff helps everyone keep things under control (stability) and allows all teammates to be apprised of what is going on with all the patients in your area (predictability).

Preceptees exhibiting predominately reactive and regard for others behaviors (Q3) are motivated primarily by social needs. Feeling connected with coworkers and creating a team spirit motivate people with reactive and responsive behaviors. As an example, suppose you work with a preceptee who exhibits predominately reactive and regard for others behaviors. This preceptee is perceived as disorganized because she is always helping other team members, so much so that she is not getting her own work done. The preceptor can influence behavior change in this situation by providing the preceptee with behavioral feedback that includes a description regarding how changing her actions would benefit the team. An example of this description would be, "I know you like to help others on the team. The best way for you to help the team is to ensure that your patient's needs are met first; then you can start helping others."

If you encounter a preceptee who is demonstrating proactive and lack of regard for others behaviors (Q1), you can influence the preceptee's behaviors by linking esteem and independence to the desired actions. For example, if you receive feedback that your preceptee is talking rudely to patient care technicians, you can make this link and influence behavior change by telling the preceptee, "I know that you value people holding you in high regard. When the technicians feel that you are talking down to them, it makes them angry. They lose respect for you, and they are hesitant to help you. In addition to derailing collaboration, continuing to demonstrate these behaviors could prolong your orientation."

If your preceptee demonstrates predominately proactive and regard for others behaviors (Q4), lucky you! When you need to influence the preceptee's behaviors, do so by linking the preceptee's independence and self-realization needs to the desired behaviors. For example, when a situation arises in which a few behavioral tweaks are needed, use feedback as a tool to help the preceptee understand how changing behaviors can lead to personal and professional growth as well as the betterment of the hospital or work area.

In summary, motivation provides the reasons underlying human behavior. Because individuals' actions broadcast their needs, using the Dimensional Model of Behavior to identify behavioral patterns can help you identify the best strategy to influence change. Preceptees exhibiting proactive and lack of regard for others behaviors are motivated by esteem and independence needs. Those preceptees exhibiting reactive and lack of regard for others behaviors are driven by security needs. Preceptees demonstrating reactive and regard for others behaviors are motivated by social needs, whereas those with predominately proactive and regard for others behaviors are driven by the need to be independent and experience growth that benefits their team.

Interacting with Influence—The Five Step Format

The Just Culture framework provides a way to shift the focus from blame to gaining insight on the factors associated with making an error. The Dimensional Model of Behavior is a tool to identify behavioral patterns of preceptees. After a behavioral pattern is identified, this information can be used to gain insight regarding how the preceptee is motivated to continue using those behaviors deemed effective and change those actions in need of an adjustment.

All of these tools can be integrated into an influence strategy that increases the odds of eliciting sustained behavior changes. The Five Step Format is a strategy that enables you to structure a conversation that influences behavior change by promoting a two-way dialogue and getting both parties involved in the discussion. This format encourages the exchange of ideas and includes formulation of an agreed-upon action plan. The five steps are:

1. Start the conversation

2. Get the preceptee's views

3. Give your views (of the preceptee's views)

4. Resolve differences

5. Develop an action plan

Step One: Start the Conversation

Starting the conversation is one of the most important parts of the interaction, because your behaviors set the tone of the conversation. As the preceptor, you possess the power, so remember that this dynamic can shut down the preceptee, especially if his or her predominant behavioral style is reactive coupled with a lack of regard for others. Starting the conversation involves appropriate sociability (which is basically a greeting) and identifying both the purpose and reason for your conversation.

Determining appropriate sociability depends upon the preceptee's primary behavior. Preceptees who primarily exhibit proactive and lack of regard for others behaviors will likely want to cut to the chase and get to the crux of the interaction. Asking this type of preceptee how his or her day is going is appropriate, but remember that this type of preceptee likes to quickly get to the task at hand. For preceptees who possesses a reactive and lack of regard for others behavioral style, too much sociability might increase their anxiety, but jumping right into the "meat of the issue" might also be a bit overwhelming. When interacting with preceptees who demonstrate predominately reactive and unresponsive behaviors, know that the conversation is going to have a slow pace and that their behavioral cues can help you sense when to increase and decrease sociability.

Preceptees with predominately reactive and regard for others behaviors require part of the interaction devoted to "social niceties," so step one is a good place for that to occur. Preceptees with predominately proactive and regard for others behaviors will engage with the social niceties and will also be prepared to discuss the situation in detail.

You can seek out the preceptee to have a discussion. Articulating up front the purpose and reason for the conversation increases both the preceptee's ownership of the issues you want to discuss and the odds that the preceptee will actively participate in the interaction. A reason tends to be focused in the past. Going back to our Just Culture examples, "I know you made a lab error last week" is an example of a reason that clarifies the behaviors that led to this interaction. Stating the purpose shifts the content of the conversation away from the past (an event the preceptee can no longer change) to the future. This shift allows the preceptor to emphasize that behavioral change is expected as the preceptee moves forward. In turn, purpose statements are most powerful when they follow reasons. Taking into account the reason scenario, an example of a purpose statement would be, "Moving forward, what kinds of things will you do to change your practice so these kinds of lab errors do not happen in the future?"

In summary, step one, starting the conversation, is your opportunity to "set the stage." Use the preceptee's predominant behavioral style as a guide to determine the appropriate level of sociability. Remember to include the reason (often an event from the past) for this conversation, as well as a purpose, which aids the dialogue in maintaining a future focus.

Step Two: Get the Preceptee's Views

Why should you get the preceptee's view of a situation before sharing your observations? Remember that as the preceptor, if you put your views "on the table" first and the preceptee does not share your opinion, the preceptee is automatically put in a defensive position because of disagreeing with you. Therefore, begin step two by asking open-ended questions. These types of questions begin with "how," "what," or "why" and invite the person to elaborate on the situation. Open-ended questions invite dialogue, and they are hard to answer with a yes or a no. Beginning step two with the example of the preceptee who mislabeled the specimen, open-ended question examples include "What are some things you will do differently in the future?" and "How will you handle multiple priorities in future situations when you are rushed?" These questions promote information sharing and can often get key points out in the open.

In essence, step two is a data-gathering exercise. Asking questions and seeking clarity are keys to the success of this step. Therefore, try to refrain from sharing your opinion at this point in the conversation (you'll get an opportunity to provide your views in step three). Preceptees with predominately reactive and lack of regard for others behaviors will likely struggle with sharing their views. Keep using open-ended questions to get at pertinent information. Pausing in between questions gives them time to respond. Preceptees who exhibit proactive and unresponsive actions or proactive and regard for others behaviors will actively participate in sharing their views. So will preceptees with predominately reactive and regard for others behaviors; in these situations, you might find yourself having to refocus the conversation. Remember that preceptees with reactive and regard for others behaviors are energized by being around people and like to talk. Closed-ended questions can help keep the conversation on topic. Closed-ended questions can be answered with a yes, no, or specific amount. Examples of closed-end questions are "Did you have a good day?" and "What is the blood pressure?" Although people often overuse closed-ended questions, they are useful when you find yourself involved in a conversation with someone who exhibits reactive and regard for others behaviors (Lefton & Buzzotta, 2004; Lefton et al., 1980). A good way to end step two is by summarizing the key points. Summary statements involve paraphrasing what you have heard and giving the preceptee the opportunity to clarify key points or areas that you might have misunderstood.

Step Three: Give Your Views (of the Preceptee's Views)

Step three provides you with the opportunity to address the information you have just received. Focus on responding to the comments you have just heard. Don't bring up feedback or information associated with the past in this step (you have time to integrate additional information in step four); the focus of step three is responding to what you just heard.

Preceptor—Mastering Difficult Conversations

- Demonstrates by openness and candor
- Has the ability to present information in a way understood by the preceptee
- Solicits the ideas of others
- Treats people with respect
- Approachable
- Focuses on accomplishing the work and engaging the preceptee

> ## Preceptor—Mastering Difficult Conversations (cont.)
>
> - Demonstrates sensitivity to the preceptee's needs
> - Promotes an effective give-and-take relationship
> - Gives constructive, actionable feedback about successes as well as developmental opportunities
> - Sparks enthusiasm
> - Challenges and involves the preceptee to see the importance of the preceptee's work and grow

Step Four: Resolve Differences

Step four can, at times, get emotional if disagreement occurs. Start off by focusing on the areas of agreement, as this sets up the ability to have a win-win situation and helps both parties ease into addressing the disagreements. If you sense the preceptee is emotional, call out those behaviors. Comments such as "You seem angry" or "You seem frustrated" can help the preceptee be candid about feelings. In turn, if anger or frustration exists, you should deal with it in the present. Having the preceptee walk away from the conversation angry or frustrated can impact the preceptee's commitment to changing behaviors. This strategy works both ways, meaning that if the preceptee senses your emotions, he or she should be comfortable enough to call out your behaviors, too.

Preceptees with reactive and lack of regard for others behaviors might struggle with sharing their emotions. When you see withdrawing behaviors, or silence, call out these behaviors because this might help preceptees express their thoughts and feelings. Preceptees with predominately reactive and regard for others behaviors are not likely to disagree, so don't let a lack of disagreement fool you into thinking they agree with you. Remember that preceptees with reactive and regard for others behaviors are motivated by acceptance so, by nature, it is hard for them to disagree with you. Preceptees with proactive and lack of regard for others or proactive and regard for others behaviors will respond to open-end questions and will share their disagreement openly.

Step Five: Developing an Action Plan

Step five plays a critical role in influencing behaviors. An effective action plan does not have to be a long document or even something in writing. Most often in precepting, the plan is a mental plan with verbalization. A plan can be a verbal agreement to touch base at the end of the shift or the next time you work together. The key to a successful action plan is creating one and following through. A plan increases the odds of follow-through and getting a commitment, whereas the lack of a plan makes it easy to slip back into old behaviors.

Conclusion

In summary, the Five Step Format is a tool you can use to organize a conversation. Each step is actually a strategy aimed at engaging the preceptee through involvement in two-way dialogue. Utilizing open-ended questions sends the message that the preceptor values the preceptee's opinion. Summary statements increase a preceptor's ability to influence behaviors, because they convey that you are listening. Allowing people to have their say and acknowledging that you heard their opinions sends the message that you value their input. Feeling valued and heard are key pieces of involvement. When people are involved, they are more likely to commit (Cialdini, 2007; Lefton & Buzzotta, 2004; Lefton et al., 1980).

In certain situations, you might encounter a preceptee who is not responding to your feedback. You might realize that even when you use these tools and put your best Q4 (proactive and regard for others) foot forward, behavioral problems remain. When these types of situations arise, assessing the fit between a preceptee and the job might be required. If you have walked the proactive and regard for others talk, sized up the preceptee's behaviors, used Just Culture to avoid attribution errors, tapped into what motivates the preceptee's actions, utilized the Five Step Format to provide candid feedback, and followed through on your action plans, then the reality might be that this preceptee is not a good match for your unit. Although these are difficult decisions to make, your actions might save the preceptee from encountering a career-ending situation.

The Just Culture provides a framework to categorize errors and omissions, whereas the Dimensional Model of Behavior helps identify specific behavioral patterns that are associated with errors. Combining a behavioral pattern assessment with the appropriate motivational links can help preceptors devise strategies of influence aimed at eliciting a sustained behavioral change.

The Five Step Format enables preceptors to engage preceptees in an active dialogue about their needs and can help preceptors gain insight regarding how preceptees view their actions. Practicing the strategies and using the tools in this chapter can help preceptors objectively identify problems and assist in providing candid and blame-free, behaviorally based feedback to the preceptees. Utilizing these strategies increases the odds that a preceptor can identify preceptor-preceptee mismatches early on and be able to guide the person to a different preceptor or to a job and environment that better match his or her clinical and people skill set.

Similar to starting an IV, delivering feedback takes practice. Just as you assess the patient's veins before you insert the IV needle, a preceptor needs to assess the preceptee before delivering feedback or attempting to influence behavior change. When solving problems related to behavior or attitude issues, attribution-free feedback based on observations sets the stage to engage preceptees in committing to change their behaviors. Regardless of the situation or the individual's behavior style, candid, blame-free feedback tailored to the individual's needs is one of the most powerful influence tools you have.

Becoming proficient at using the Dimensional Model of Behavior, the Just Culture framework, the Behavioral Pyramid, and the Five Step Format takes practice. Combining your clinical mastery with people skills enables you to impact patient care through others. Using proactive and regard for others strategies to help the preceptee grow is a journey. The journey involves role-modeling the behaviors you expect from others and providing blame-free, objective, observational-based feedback that motivates the preceptee to strive for excellence in both clinical and people skills.

References

Aiken, L. H., Clarke, S. P., Sloane, D. M., Lake, E. T., & Cheney, T. (2008). Effects of hospital care environments on patient mortality and nurse outcomes. *Journal of Nursing Administration (JONA)*, *38*(5), 223-229.

American Association of Critical-Care Nurses (2005). AACN Standards for establishing and sustaining healthy work environments: A journey to excellence. *American Journal of Critical Care*, 14(3), 187-197.

Cialdini, R. B. (2007). *Influence: The psychology of persuasion*. New York, NY: HarperCollins Publishers.

GAIN Working Group E, Flight Ops/ATC Ops Safety Information Sharing. (2004). *A roadmap to a Just Culture: Enhancing the safety environment*. Retrieved from http://www.nmhanet.org/work-force/just-culture/Roadmap%20to%20a%20Just%20Culture-GAIN.pdf

Gilbert, D. T., & Malone, P. S. (1995). The correspondence bias. *Psychological Bulletin*, *117*(1), 21-38.

Hall, C. S., & Lindzey, G. (1979). *Theories of personality*. Hoboken, NJ: John Wiley & Sons.

Heider, F. (1958). *The psychology of interpersonal relations*. New York: John Wiley & Sons.

Kohn, L. T., Corrigan, J. M., & Donaldson, M. S., (Eds.). (2000). *To err is human*. Institute of Medicine. Washington, DC: National Academy Press.

Lefton, R. E., & Buzzotta, V. R. (2004). *Leadership through people skills*. New York, NY: McGraw-Hill.

Lefton, R. E., Buzzotta, V. R., & Sherberg, M. (1980). *Improving productivity through people skills: Dimensional management strategies*. Cambridge, MA: Ballinger Publishing Company.

Marx, D. (2008). *Just culture: Training for healthcare managers* (4th ed.). Plano, TX: Outcome Engineering, LLC.

Perlini, A. H., & Ward, C. (2000). HIV prevention interventions: The effects of role-play and behavioural commitment on knowledge and attitudes. *Canadian Journal of Behavioural Science, 32*(3), 133-143.

Petrocelli, J. V., Clarkson, J. J., Tormala, Z. L., & Hendrix, K. S. (2010). Perceiving stability as a means to attitude certainty: The role of implicit theories of attitude. *Journal of Experimental Social Psychology, 46*(6), 874-883. doi: 10.1016/j.jesp.2010.07.012

Potter, P., Wolf, L., Boxerman, S., Grayson, D., Sledge, J., Dunagan, C., & Evanoff, B. (2005). An analysis of nurses' cognitive work: A new perspective for understanding medical errors. In K. Henriksen, J. B. Battles, E. S. Marks, & D. I. Lewin (Eds.) (pp. 39-51). *Advances in patient safety: From research to implementation, 1.*Rockville, MD. Agency for Healthcare Research and Quality.

Preceptor Development Plan
Assessing and Addressing Preceptee Behavior and Motivation

Review the information on assessing and addressing preceptee behavior and motivation described in this chapter. What are your strengths? In which areas do you need to increase your knowledge and expertise? What is your plan for expanding your knowledge and expertise? What resources are available? Who can help you?

What is the predominant way of dealing with behavior and errors in your organization? If it is not a Just Culture, what can you do to influence the use of Just Culture with your preceptee?

Think about your own behavior and motivation. What is your predominant behavior? What motivates you?

Name:			
Just Culture			
Strengths	Needs	Plan	Resources
Providing Feedback			
Strengths	Needs	Plan	Resources
Behavior			
Strengths	Needs	Plan	Resources
Motivation			
Strengths	Needs	Plan	Resources
Influence			
Strengths	Needs	Plan	Resources

Note: This form and other resources are available at www.RNPreceptor.com.

Pragmatics of Precepting

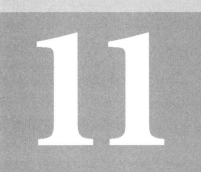

Larissa Marquez Africa, MBA, BSN, RN
Cherilyn Ashlock, MSN, RN

Preceptors have the enormous responsibility of ensuring that preceptees under their wings are not only clinically competent, but also exude the values of the profession and the organization. Preceptees look to preceptors as role models on providing safe, competent care. This chapter discusses the pragmatics of precepting, including strategies and techniques preceptors can use to assist preceptees with organization, time management, and delegation; strategies on how to manage challenges with preceptees' clinical skill development; and strategies on how to manage negative and unproductive behaviors.

Organization and Time Management

How do preceptors organize the duties of the precepting role while at the same time providing patient care with preceptees, knowing that—as preceptors—their behavior is constantly being observed by preceptees who see them as role models? How do preceptees learn to organize and manage their own time? Time management and organization skills are critical for efficient, productive nursing practice, but they are often the most difficult to teach. Strategies and techniques for organization and time management should be embedded into all areas of precepting, including preparation for the shift and patient assignment, the shift report, the preceptor

OBJECTIVES

- Utilize strategies and techniques to assist in the preceptee's organization, time management, and delegation skill development

- Apply strategies on how to manage challenges with preceptee's clinical skill development

- Manage negative and unproductive preceptee behaviors

and preceptee shift, and the overall orientation experience for the nurse, which includes establishing a routine for delivery of care.

Preparing for the Shift and Patient Assignment

The role of the preceptor in preparation for the daily shift includes ensuring the appropriate assignment, advocating for the preceptee's learning experience, and preparing for educational opportunities. Preceptors need to arrive early for the shift to allow time to meet with the charge nurse and request an appropriate assignment. If the preceptee needs to work on a specific skill or particular type of patient diagnosis or procedure, look for those types of patients and request that assignment. Often a preceptor is forced into a circumstance where the shift assignment is "overloaded" because of the perception that the preceptor and preceptee are two nurses and can carry a heavier patient load. Determine whether the assignment is unrealistic and does not resemble a typical nursing care assignment. Similar to how a nurse advocates for patients, the preceptor should also serve as an advocate for the preceptee.

Shift Report

Shift report or patient handoff is crucial to the development of the preceptee. Shift report should be the foundation for the organization of the shift for both the preceptor and the preceptee. Shift report can be a foreign concept to new graduate nurses and even experienced nurses who have learned a different method from past experiences. The process of participating in a shift report can be intimidating to a new nurse on the unit, and easing the preceptee into the process is helpful. During the first days of precepting, allow the preceptee to observe shift to shift report. As the preceptee's clinical experience progresses, ask the preceptee to document the report in preparation for delivery to oncoming staff. A practice or role-play of delivering a shift report might alleviate some of the anxiety the preceptee is experiencing. Provide feedback to the preceptee as soon as possible.

The Preceptor and Preceptee Shift

Styles of precepting that foster clinical decision-making and assist in the transition of a nurse to independent practice can vary. The traditional method of precepting encourages a preceptee to follow the style, delivery of care, and organization of the preceptor. The preceptee follows and takes direction from the preceptor as the delivery of care for the patient assignment is provided. The preceptee observes the interaction and patient education that occurs during the shift. If the preceptee is struggling with a particular concept or skill, consider a half or full shift of focused care delivery. For example, if the preceptee needs to hone in on skills surrounding physical assessment and documentation, consider having the preceptee spend the first few hours of the shift performing a head-to-toe assessment and documenting observations on the organization's documentation system or chart.

Establishing a Routine and Facilitating Prioritization

To effectively precept, you need to establish a routine and assist the preceptee in prioritizing patient care. At the beginning of each shift, clearly define what needs to be accomplished together. The preceptor should help the preceptee prioritize a plan of care for the day based on the needs of the patient assignment. One system of prioritization encourages the nurse to rank tasks based on the CURE scale:

- **C**—critical; potentially life threatening
- **U**—urgent; safety needs, pain control, anything that could potentially cause harm or discomfort for the patient
- **R**—routine; scheduled shift activities
- **E**—extra; comfort requests of the patient (Nelson et al., 2006)

The CURE strategy assists with task mastery. As soon as task mastery is no longer an obstacle, the preceptee can see the bigger picture. After a prioritized plan has been established, the preceptor and preceptee should continue to communicate, reevaluate, and reprioritize throughout the day and as needs arise. The preceptee might find that breaking the shift into small increments of time and setting overall goals are useful strategies in organizing the day. A daily organization sheet (see Table 11.1 for an example) is often useful in helping the preceptee establish a routine. At some point during the shift, set aside time for reflection, feedback, and documentation of competency acquisition and future goal setting.

Table 11.1   Sample Daily Organization Sheet. (Adapt as needed for different shifts or time frames.)

Daily Organization Cheat Sheet

0700-0800
- Shift report
- Prepare/organize plan of care for day; complete cheat sheet

0800-0900
- Check vital signs on all patients and delegate tasks to assistive personnel
- Physical assessment and documentation—312, 313, 314, 317

0900-1000
- Medications—312, 313, 317
- Check a.m. labs on all patients
- Break

1000-1100
- Medications—314
- Check for new orders on all patients

1100-1200
- Pt reassessment and documentation

1200-1300
- Medications—314, 315
- Lunch

1300-1400
- Care plan and education documentation for all patients
- Prepare patient in room 317 for cath lab

1400-1500
- Anticipated surgery admission, room 315
- Cath lab procedure scheduled—317

1500-1600
- Admission assessment—315
- Check admission orders and prepare paperwork/chart for continued care of admission

1600-1700
- Family care conference—314
- Break

1700-1800
- Ensure documentation on all patients is up to date
- Reflection and feedback with preceptor
- Documentation of competencies with preceptor

1800-1900
- Prepare for shift report
- Room clean-up and prep for next shift

Delegation

Following the development of a prioritized plan for the day/shift, the next step is delegation. The National Council of State Boards of Nursing (NCSBN; 1995, p. 2) defines *delegation* as "Transferring to a competent individual the authority to perform a selected nursing task in a selected situation." The nurse retains accountability for the delegation.

Delegation is one of the most complex skills to teach a preceptee—what the preceptee can delegate and to whom, and what can be delegated to the preceptee. Preceptors also need to help new graduate nurse preceptees understand that they cannot do everything themselves and that they need to delegate tasks when possible, to have time to perform the patient care that only RNs are qualified to do.

Weydt (2010) notes that effective delegation is based on the state nurse practice act as well as an understanding of the concepts of responsibility, authority, and accountability. In addition, the American Nurses Association (ANA) and the NCSBN (2006, p. 3), in a joint statement on delegation, note that "the effective use of delegation requires a nurse to have a body of practice experience and the authority to implement delegation."

The delegation process, as described by the NCSBN (1995), includes the following:

- Understand delegation criteria—what is allowed under the state nurse practice act, qualifications of the delegator and scope of authority to delegate, qualifications of the delegatee.

- Assess the situation—needs of the patient, circumstances, availability of resources including supervision.

- Plan for the task to be delegated—nature of the task and knowledge and skills required to perform it, competence of delegatee, implications.

- Assure accountability—delegator and delegatee.

- Supervise performance of the task—provide directions and expectations, monitor performance, intervene if needed, ensure documentation.

- Evaluate the delegation process—patient, performance of task.

- Reassess and adjust as needed.

Assuring competence in delegation is important for all preceptees, but especially for new graduate nurses who may not have had the opportunity to delegate during their student experience. The preceptor must first assess the competence of the preceptee to delegate, assuring that the preceptee can perform all the functions of the delegation process. Gaps in preceptee competence must then be filled by developing the preceptee's knowledge and skills as needed. When the preceptee is competent, the preceptor can begin to work with the preceptee on a daily basis to determine what tasks can be delegated that day and to whom, and to effectively use all components of the delegation process.

Principles of Delegation—American Nurses Association

Overarching Principles

- The nursing profession determines the scope of nursing practice.

- The nursing profession defines and supervises the education, training and utilization for any assistant roles involved in providing direct patient care.

- The RN takes responsibility and accountability for the provision of nursing practice.

- The RN directs care and determines the appropriate utilization of any assistant involved in providing direct patient care.

- The RN accepts aid from nursing assistive personnel in providing nursing care for the patient.

Nurse-Related Principles

- The RN takes responsibility and accountability for the provision of nursing practice.

- The RN directs care and determines the appropriate utilization of any assistant involved in providing direct patient care.

- The RN may delegate components of care but does not delegate the nursing process itself. The practice pervasive functions of assessment, planning, evaluation and nursing judgment cannot be delegated.

- The decision of whether or not to delegate or assign is based upon the RN's judgment concerning the condition of the patient, the competence of all members of the nursing team and the degree of supervision that will be required of the RN if a task is delegated.

- The RN delegates only those tasks for which she or he believes the other health care worker has the knowledge and skill to perform, taking into consideration training, cultural competence, experience and facility/agency policies and procedures.

- The RN individualizes communication regarding the delegation to the nursing assistive personnel and client situation and the communication should be clear, concise, correct and complete. The RN verifies comprehension with the nursing assistive personnel and that the assistant accepts the delegation and the responsibility that accompanies it.

- Communication must be a two-way process. Nursing assistive personnel should have the opportunity to ask questions and/or for clarification of expectations.

- The RN uses critical thinking and professional judgment when following the Five Rights of Delegation, to be sure that the delegation or assignment is:

  - The right task

  - Under the right circumstances

  - To the right person

  - With the right directions and communication; and

  - Under the right supervision and evaluation.

- Chief Nursing Officers are accountable for establishing systems to assess, monitor, verify and communicate ongoing competence requirements in areas related to delegation.

- There is both individual accountability and organizational accountability for delegation. Organizational accountability for delegation relates to providing sufficient resources, including:

  - Sufficient staffing with an appropriate staff mix

  - Documenting competencies for all staff providing direct patient care and for ensuring that the RN has access to competence information for the staff to whom the RN is delegating care

  - Organizational policies on delegation are developed with the active participation of all nurses, and acknowledge that delegation is a professional right and responsibility.

Organization Principles

- The organization is accountable for delegation through the allocation of resources to ensure sufficient staffing so that the RN can delegate appropriately.

- The organization is accountable for documenting competencies for all staff providing direct patient care and for ensuring that the RN has access to competency information for staff to whom the RN is delegating patient care.

Principles of Delegation—American Nurses Association (cont.)

- Organizational policies on delegation are developed with the active participation of all nurses (staff, managers and administrators).

- The organization ensures that the educational needs of nursing assistive personnel are met through the implementation of a system that allows for nurse input.

- Organizations have policies in place that allow input from nurses indicating that delegation is a professional right and responsibility.

Source: ANA, 2005

Performance Discrepancies

A performance discrepancy occurs when there is a difference between what is and what should be—a difference between actual performance and expected performance (Mager & Pipe, 1997). Effectively resolving a performance discrepancy requires the use of a systematic process that begins with identifying the discrepancy. While it is often tempting to think you know the problem when you first identify the discrepancy, experience teaches that things are not always what they seem.

Mager and Pipe (1997) have described the components of analyzing and resolving performance discrepancies:

- Describe the problem. Make sure you fully and accurately understand the problem.

  - What is the performance discrepancy? What is the actual performance at issue? What is the desired performance?

  - Is it worth pursuing? For example, the preceptee does a patient assessment in a different order than you've demonstrated. It's different, but does the order really matter? What would happen if you left it alone? Are your expectations reasonable? What are the consequences caused by the discrepancy?

- Explore fast fixes (obvious solutions).

  - Can you apply fast fixes? Does the preceptee know what is expected? Can the preceptee describe the desired performance and the expected accomplishments? Are there obvious obstacles to the desired performance? Does the preceptee get regular feedback on performance?

- Check the consequences.

  - Is the desired performance punishing? What are the consequences of performing as desired? Is it actually punishing or perceived as punishing?

  - Is the undesired performance rewarding in any way? For example, does the preceptee get more attention from you when doing the undesired performance? What rewards, prestige, status, or comfort support the present way of doing things? Does misbehaving get more attention than doing it right?

  - Are there any consequences at all? Does the desired performance lead to consequences that the preceptee sees as favorable?

- Enhance competence.

  - Is it a skill deficiency? Could the preceptee do it if he or she really had to?

  - Could the preceptee do it in the past? If yes, what changed?

  - Is the skill used often? How often is the performance displayed? How often is the skill applied?

  - Is there regular feedback on how things are going?

  - Can the task be simplified? Are all the requirements necessary? Can you provide the preceptee with performance aids? Can you redesign the workplace or provide physical help?

  - Are there any obstacles remaining? Does something get in the way of doing it right? Is there a lack of knowledge about what is expected? Are there conflicting demands or restrictive policies?

  - Does the preceptee have what it takes to do the job? Is it likely that the preceptee can learn to do the task? Does the preceptee lack the physical or mental potential to perform as desired?

- Develop solutions.

  - Which solution is best? Have all potential solutions been identified? Does each solution identified address one or more parts of the problem? What are the tangible and intangible costs of each potential solution? Which solutions are the most practical, feasible, and economical? Which yield the most value, solving the largest part of the problem(s) for the least effort?

- Implement solutions and reassess.

It is important for the preceptor to identify and address preceptee performance discrepancies as soon as possible. Using this process, the preceptor can determine the real problem(s) and can work with the preceptee to create one or more solutions that resolve the discrepancy.

Problem Solving Preceptor-Preceptee Relationships

The preceptor is key to the success of a preceptee's clinical immersion. But, what happens when the preceptee has difficulty learning the clinical skills or is displaying behavior not conducive to learning? What if the preceptor-preceptee match is just not working?

When Skill Development Becomes a Challenge

The preceptor role-models safe, competent patient care and demonstrates the realities of practice for the preceptee (Barker & Pittman, 2010). When skill development becomes a challenge, a preceptor might consider the following:

- Clarify the overall goals and goals for each clinical shift.

- Solicit assistance of others in the department, such as the charge nurse, to ensure that the preceptee can get the experience.

- Provide constructive feedback.

Clarifying Clinical Goals

Communicating the clinical goals not only is essential in organizing the plan of care for the day, but also assists in clarifying what needs to be achieved overall and during each shift. Goals should be realistic and concise, and have an identified time frame. The goals should be written, if possible, and discussed with the preceptee. The preceptee should be given a copy of the documented goals. Whether the competency being evaluated is technical, interpersonal, behavioral, or critical thinking, the key is giving "clear guidelines regarding competency expectations" (Swihart, 2007, p. 17).

Appropriate Patient Care Assignments

Validating clinical competencies can be a challenge if the patient care assignment is not appropriate or does not match the competency that needs to be validated. Soliciting assistance from other nurses on the unit and the charge nurse can help ensure that the preceptee receives the clinical experience he or she needs. For example, if the preceptee is having difficulty with central venous catheter care after repeated instructions and demonstration, the charge nurse might be able to identify other patients in the department who need central venous catheter care. Barker and Pittman (2010) suggest that matching patients and learners for a specific learning experience is one of the effective techniques of precepting.

The preceptor should assist the preceptee in understanding the low-frequency, high-risk skills development. If a patient on the unit is utilizing a piece of equipment or experiencing a procedure, advocate for the preceptee to be exposed to this experience, even if it is not part of the preceptee-preceptor assignment. Most importantly, the preceptor should focus the majority of the onboarding time on preparing the new nurse for a realistic post-onboarding assignment. For example, if the nurses on the unit typically start the shift with five patients, discharge one, and take two admissions, most of the clinical onboarding shifts should look similar to this scenario. If most of the patients on the unit have a certain diagnosis or group of diagnoses, most of the preceptee and preceptor assignments should prepare the nurse to care for that patient population.

Providing Feedback

Providing specific, constructive feedback is essential for the preceptee's learning. Providing feedback does not have to begin at the end of the skill that the preceptee is asked to demonstrate. Providing feedback can begin the moment the preceptor asks the preceptee to demonstrate the task. Beginning the feedback process early encourages independent thinking and allows the connection between prior knowledge and practice knowledge, thus empowering the preceptee to critically think (Sorensen & Yankech, 2008). Some strategies for providing feedback are shown in Table 11.2.

Table 11.2   Strategies for Providing Feedback

- Provide a specific description of what you had observed. Statements such as "You did an excellent job of . . ." are helpful.
- Focus on sharing information rather than giving advice. Statements such as "Many times when . . ." teach general rules.
- Provide feedback in a timely manner, and avoid providing feedback where everyone can hear the conversation. Questions such as "What do you think is going on?" or "What led you to that conclusion?" can assist in formulating the feedback to the preceptee.
- Give enough time for feedback to be accepted prior to making a plan for future validation.
- Avoid giving the impression that you and other staff members are "ganging up" on your preceptee.

Challenging Behaviors

"Success is the result of the positive work habits we form and observe on a daily basis" (Joseph & Lakshmi, 2011, p. 43). The negative impact of unacceptable behaviors can affect productivity and decision-making processes (Appelbaum & Shapiro, 2006; Brinkert, 2010). Clearly identifying the specifics is essential before the behavior that hinders the learning process can be managed. Similar to the importance of focusing on behaviors when providing feedback on skill development, identify and document the behaviors considered unacceptable. Behaviors also include nonverbal cues such as eye rolling and crossing of arms across the chest. Documentation of how frequently the behaviors are displayed can help summarize the information for the discussion.

The goal is to be prepared to explain to the preceptee the cause of concern and the reason why an immediate change in behavior is necessary (Grote, 2005). Reasons why an immediate change is necessary might include the impact of the inappropriate behavior toward coworkers, patients, and families; values and standards of the organization; and a negative impact on the learning process. Just as feedback on the preceptee's clinical competencies is best given in a safe environment, addressing negative behaviors is also best given in a safe, private environment. As Grote (2005) suggests, "Discuss the situation with the individual and explain that his behavior—not his attitude—is causing a problem." Provide information on the specific behaviors observed. Discuss the rationale for why the behaviors are of concern and ask for help in solving the problem. Denial might be the initial response from the preceptee. The goal is to communicate the problem and ensure that a plan to address the issue is in place if it cannot be solved at that moment.

Preceptor-Preceptee Mismatch

A successful preceptor-preceptee relationship can rely on several factors. Sometimes, preceptors are told they are going to be preceptors instead of being asked if they want to be preceptors. According to Barker and Pittman (2010), the nurse must agree to be a preceptor and should have some knowledge and understanding of the roles and responsibilities of precepting. Matching teaching styles with learning styles has also been cited as an important factor when matching preceptors with preceptees (Vaughn & Baker, 2008). Unfortunately, even if these factors are taken into consideration, the preceptor-preceptee relationship might not be successful. Forcing the preceptor-preceptee relationship even after attempts to address the challenges of skill development and negative behaviors can negatively impact the preceptor's experience and the success of the preceptee. At this point, the manager should be involved in the discussions. The preceptor-preceptee-manager discussion should occur in an attempt to resolve the situation. If either the preceptor or preceptee is not finding any benefit to the relationship, the manager should reassign the preceptee with another preceptor. The mismatch might be a result of simple differences in personalities. The preceptee might struggle with one preceptor, but thrive with another. This is not a reflection of the preceptor or preceptee's performance, but just a mismatch of the relationship.

Conclusion

Preceptors face many challenges in their role. This chapter is designed to provide useful tools and words of anticipation to help preceptors prepare for common mishaps. A key to successfully transitioning a new nurse from onboarding to independent practice requires an assessment of the preceptee's organizational and time management skills, use of the tools to bridge the gap, goal setting, and providing timely feedback to achieve clinical competence. Finally, the preceptor needs to confront challenging behaviors and correct preceptor-preceptee mismatches to ensure the success of both the preceptor and preceptee.

References

American Nurses Association (ANA). (2005). *Principles for delegation.* Silver Spring, MD: Author.

American Nurses Association (ANA) and National Council of State Boards of Nursing (NCSBN). (2006). *Joint statement on delegation.* Retrieved from https://www.ncsbn.org/pdfs/Joint_statement.pdf

Appelbaum, S. H., & Shapiro, B. T. (2006). Diagnosis and remedies for deviant workplace behaviors. *Journal of American Academy of Business, Cambridge, 9*(2), 14-20.

Barker, E. R., & Pittman, O. (2010). Becoming a super preceptor: A practical guide to preceptorship in today's clinical climate. *Journal of the American Academy of Nurse Practitioners, 22*(3), 144-149.

Brinkert, R. (2010). A literature review of conflict communication causes, costs, benefits, and interventions in nursing. *Journal of Nursing Management, 18*(2), 145-156.

Grote, D. (2005, July). Attitude adjustments: To deal with an employee's bad attitude, focus on his or her specific behaviors. *HR Magazine, 50*(7). Retrieved from http://findarticles.com/p/articles/mi_m3495/is_7_50/ai_n14814551/

Joseph, C., & Lakshmi, S. S. (2011). Developing positive habits in the workplace. *The IUP Journal of Soft Skills, V*(1), 37-44.

Mager, R.F. & Pipe, P. (1997). *Analyzing performance problems: Or, you really gotta wanna. How to figure out why people aren't doing what they should be, and what to do about it.* Atlanta, GA: The Center for Effective Performance, Inc.

National Council of State Boards of Nursing (NCSBN). (1995). *Delegation: Concepts and decision-making process. National Council Position Paper.* Chicago, IL: Author.

Nelson, J. L., Kummeth, P. J., Crane, L. J., Mueller, C. L., Olson, C. J., Schatz, T. F., & Wilson, D. M. (2006). Teaching prioritization skills: A preceptor forum. *Journal for Nurses in Staff Development, 22*, 172-178. Retrieved from http://www.biomedsearch.com/nih/Teaching-prioritization-skills-preceptor-forum/16885681.html

Sorensen, H. A., & Yankech, L. R. (2008). Precepting in the fast lane: Improving critical thinking in new graduate nurses. *The Journal of Continuing Education in Nursing, 39*(5), 208-216.

Swihart, D. (2007). *The effective nurse preceptor handbook: Your guide to success* (2nd ed.). Marblehead, MA: HCPro, Inc.

Vaughn, L. M., & Baker, R. (2008). Do different pairings of teaching styles and learning styles make a difference? Preceptor and resident perceptions. *Teaching and Learning in Medicine, 20*(3), 239-247.

Weydt, A. (2010, May 31). Developing delegation skills. *OJIN: The Online Journal of Issues in Nursing, 15*(2), Manuscript 1.

Preceptor Development Plan: Pragmatics of Precepting

Review the information on pragmatics of precepting described in this chapter. What are your strengths? In which areas do you need to increase your knowledge and expertise? What is your plan for expanding your knowledge and expertise? What resources are available? Who can help you?

Name:			
Organization and Time Management			
Strengths	Needs	Plan	Resources
Problem Solving Preceptor-Preceptee Relationships			
Strengths	Needs	Plan	Resources
Challenging Behaviors			
Strengths	Needs	Plan	Resources
Motivation			
Strengths	Needs	Plan	Resources
Influence			
Strengths	Needs	Plan	Resources

Note: This form and other resources are available at www.RNPreceptor.com.

"Leadership and learning are indispensable to each other."

–John Fitzgerald Kennedy

For Managers: Selecting, Supporting, and Sustaining Preceptors

12

Carol A. Bradley, MSN, RN, CENP
Amy K. Doepken, BSN, RN, CCRN
Denise D. Fall, BSN, RN
Mary L. Feldt, MSN, RN
Jennifer L. Thornburgh, BSN, RN
Collista J. Zook, MS, CNS, RN

OBJECTIVES

- Utilize standard concepts in the development of preceptor performance standards

- Compose standardized, objective tools for preceptor selection and evaluation

- Assemble developmental and supportive processes for the preceptor role

- Identify creative strategies for sustaining and overcoming challenges in preceptor programs

Selecting, supporting, and sustaining a skilled workforce begin with a sound preceptor program. A team approach is essential to the successful development of nurses and their integration into the organization and their units/departments. The nurse manager has the unique opportunity to create an environment of growth and development for newly hired nurses, new nurse graduates, and current staff seeking to expand clinical and leadership skills through a sustainable precepting program. Developing uniform selection criteria, establishing performance standards, successfully matching preceptors and preceptees, supporting education, utilizing evaluation as a means for growth, providing meaningful recognition, and utilizing creative solutions to overcome challenges are key components to incorporate in successfully developing a comprehensive preceptor program. A strong preceptor program will foster a collaborative, engaged, and sustainable workforce.

Establishing Performance Standards

Performance standards provide the fundamental structure by which nursing practice is defined by national and specialty agencies. These standards can be broad in scope, applying to all nurses, or narrowed to a specific clinical practice. Professional organizations establish nursing performance standards. The American Nurses Association provides a nursing code of ethics (ANA, 2001) and standards of practice (ANA, 2010). Organizations should use the code and standards as a starting point for developing their individual performance standards. Specialty areas should rely on established professional standards of commitment to patients, advocacy, and accountability for nursing practice (for example, American Association of Critical-Care Nurses [AACN], Association of periOperative Registered Nurses [AORN], Emergency Nurses Association [ENA], and Oncology Nursing Society [ONS]). Professional behaviors based on performance standards are the cornerstone for establishing objective evaluative criteria for all employees' performance. These standards should promote effective patient care, including patient rights and safety, patient- and family-centered care, patient education, clinical judgment, interpersonal communication, information management, and professional development. Integrating individual health care organizational values with national and professional bodies is essential in guiding the development of preceptor performance standards. An example of preceptor standards of a development model from Legacy Health is shown in Figure 12.1.

Defining successful outcomes for preceptors is the next step in creating a strong preceptor program. A successful program promotes the independent, competent practice of a nurse. Nursing units need to establish formal criteria for the completion of their orientation programs. Establishing performance goals clearly communicates expectations. A template you can use to clearly communicate required expectations indicative of successful skill acquisition for nurses being precepted in various roles and clinical settings is shown in Table 12.1. Populate the cells with the desired outcomes.

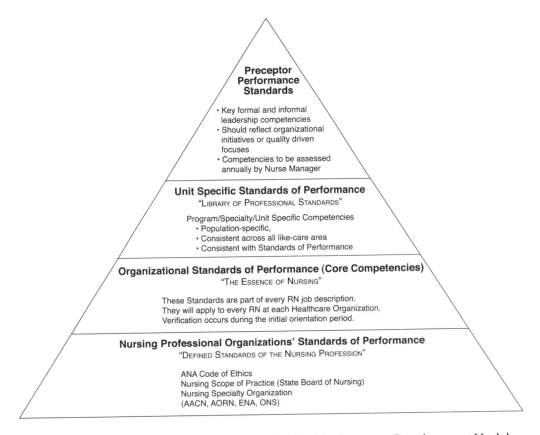

Figure 12.1   Legacy Health Preceptor Standards of Performance Development Model

Table 12.1 Defining Successful Outcomes			
	Clinical Ability	*Problem-Solving Ability*	*Communication & Patient Advocacy*
New Hire			
New Graduate Nurse			
Transitioning Nurse			
Experienced Specialty Nurse			
Clinical Advancement for Current Nurse			
Other			

Demonstration of competency defines successful completion of onboarding. Checklists or passive education modalities cannot measure competency. Establish competencies for clinical ability, problem-solving ability, and communication skills. Timelines for successful completion should be flexible and depend upon the preceptor and preceptee's skill level.

Developing the Foundation—Preceptor Selection Criteria

The process for selecting preceptors can vary immensely and be characterized by an inconsistent application of selection criteria. In the majority of clinical settings, preceptor selection is based on seniority in the unit or expertise (Beecroft, Hernandez, & Reid, 2008). For managers, utilization of this widely used selection criteria can become problematic because of unclear expectations for preceptors and lack of blending organizational values into the selection process. This inconsistent approach also makes it impossible to develop resource tools to assist managers with their decision-making for preceptor selection.

Selection criteria for preceptors must be clearly defined to ensure that application to standards is uniform for each nurse. Clear, definitive selection criteria can help establish consistency and a more formalized process to select preceptors. First, blending organizational values with unit-specific needs is essential to development of the preceptor criteria. "There must be careful preplanning on the part of all stakeholders who must be committed to the program, from administrators to managers to preceptors, as well as the other staff. The mission, purpose, goals, and outcomes of the program must be clearly documented" (Myrick & Yonge, 2005, p. 142).

To best represent your precepting criteria, combine your organization's mission and values with unit/department-specific skill needs. Key attributes to consider from your organizational values might include developing lines of communication, staying open to feedback, displaying a positive attitude, creating professional behaviors, meeting clinical performance standards, developing confidence to advocate for patient and family needs, demonstrating the ability to work in a team, developing motivation to teach others, and participating in active role-modeling in supporting the organization's mission.

By blending organizational values with unit-specific standards, you can establish a "core" of standards. Nurse preceptors must then meet these organizational core performance standards. As an example, Legacy Health in Portland, Oregon, uses its Preferred Employee Profile as the minimum expectation of organizational core performance standards. Legacy Health's values—do the right thing, be a team player, respect each other, provide exceptional service, deliver outstanding quality, commit to excellence, take responsibility, embrace innovation, and lead the way (see Figure 12.2)—become a portion of the organizational core performance standards to be a preceptor.

Preferred Employee Profile

Expectations for Legacy Employees

Highly skilled and committed employees are critical to Legacy's success. We set high expectations, and hold our employees accountable to act consistently with the core values that drive our mission. We exemplify our values through the following actions:

Do the Right Thing Model a high standard of conduct, honesty, and integrity in all situations. Act responsibly with sensitive and private information. Respect patients' and co-workers' rights to confidentiality. Comply with all legal and regulatory compliance standards.

Be a Team Player Build productive relationships. Communicate effectively, surface and resolve conflict, listen actively and solicit feedback. Encourage cooperation, develop trust and support teammates.

Respect Others Always communicate to others in a professional, respectful and kind manner. Demonstrate a welcoming and inclusive environment for our employees, patients and visitors. Embrace and celebrate our differences and similarities.

Provide Exceptional Service Put patients and their families at the center of all work activities. Exceed internal and external customers' expectations and anticipate needs. Take the time to ensure external and internal customers feel valued. Respond constructively and positively to customer issues.

Deliver Outstanding Quality Consistently deliver outstanding quality of service and patient care. Strive to improve work processes and outcomes. Meet standards, use data and measure results for constant improvement. Participate actively in reducing errors, eliminating waste and assuring patient safety.

Commit to Excellence Set high standards of performance for yourself and others to achieve exceptional results. Commit to personal and professional development and continual learning. Adopt best practices and actively engage in improvement efforts.

Take Responsibility Keep your commitments. Openly admit mistakes. Be accountable for your actions and decisions and for department and organizational success. Be a good steward of organizational resources.

Embrace Innovation Actively engage in new initiatives, learn and adopt new work methods, and embrace change in a positive productive manner. Seek opportunities to test ideas, think progressively and question the status quo.

Lead the Way Be a role model for excellent performance, high quality work, respectful communication, teamwork, and exceptional service.

LEGACY
HEALTH

HR-4279

Figure 12.2   Legacy Health Preferred Employee Profile
Source: Legacy Health. Copyrighted. Used with permission.

After the nurse manager observes that nurses meet the organizational core performance standards, an integrated classification tool can assist in determining preceptors' potential. Legacy Health also developed a nursing preceptor rubric that allows the manager to quantify and classify a preceptor's capability utilizing a rubric format and Patricia Benner's novice to expert theory (Benner, 1984; see Figure 12.3). Use of the rubric establishes consistency and eliminates variation of standards in the selection process.

LEGACY
HEALTH

Nursing Preceptor Rubric

Name _____ Date _____ Medical Center/Unit _____
  Q Check box if Preceptor Candidate will be Precepting in the Nurse Residency Program

All Legacy nurses must meet all of the preferred Employee Profile Criteria to be eligible to be a preceptor.

Patricia Benner, RN, PhD is a nursing theorist who patented her Novice-to-Expert Theory to explain a nurse's development process. There are five levels of nursing experience: Novice, Advanced Beginner, Competent, Proficient, and Expert. The spectrum shows the progression from brand new nurse who thinks everything through in steps, to a nurse who is able to practice intuitively. Benner's Novice to Expert theory is now the basis for precepting at Legacy. A sequential progression of nurses from the Competent, Proficient and then Expert level will be utilized during the orientation process. We need to clearly identify what category each of our preceptor is in. All criteria must be met in each box to receive that designation.

Criteria	Competent level Column #1	Proficient level Column #2	Expert level Column #3
Demonstrate Accountability	☐ Some experience on which to build nursing judgments. Has developed baseline advocacy skills for the patient and family. Demonstrates basic skills & knowledge. Explains basic rationale for interventions, processes, and plans. Performs conscious, deliberate planning which results in efficiency and organization. Possesses the basic ability to prioritize appropriately. Has his/her own style of nursing practice based on evidence-based practice. Is knowledgeable about and willingly to utilizes resources Adheres to organization & department policies. Can see the whole picture, but may need support to achieve all the desired patient outcomes. May need assistance individualizing patients care plan	☐ Has substantial experience in patient care and exhibits sound clinical judgment. Advanced advocacy skills for the patient and family Demonstrates skills in the recognition of situational changes requiring unplanned and unanticipated interventions. More in-depth understanding of rational for interventions, processes, and plans. Succinctly plans, advocates and initiates individualized plan of care for patients. Able to effectively prioritize. Exemplifies evidence-based nursing practice. Readily accesses and uses resources. Can reference policies in daily practice and during emergencies Independently able to achieve the desired patient outcomes. Independently able to individualized each patient's care plan.	☐ An experienced nurse who functions as a role model in their unit. Exceptional advocacy skills for the patient and family Possesses comprehensive knowledge & skills. Exceptional understanding of rational for interventions, processes, and plans. Easily manages the most complex situations and can disseminate that knowledge to others. Models evidence- base practice, leadership skills and high-level conflict resolution abilities. Readily evaluates practice against organization & department policies. He/she instrumental as a change agent for evidence based practice. Excellent skill in developing care plan to support desired outcomes. Expert with individualizing patient's care plan to meet their needs.

Figure 12.3   Legacy Health Nursing Preceptor Rubric
Source: Legacy Health. Copyrighted. Used with permission.

Criteria	Competent level Column #1	Proficient level Column #2	Expert level Column #3
Manage for Excellence	☐ Needs lots of support to develop plan for their preceptee. May need assistance with coaching preceptee.	☐ Needs minimal support to develop plan for preceptee. Developing ability to coach preceptee.	☐ Able to independently establish learning plan and discern preceptee's ability. Can successfully coach preceptee.
Emphasize Teamwork	☐ Is willing to serve as a preceptor. Able to contribute to the team effort by assisting peers and members of the healthcare team at times. May need mentor for providing care	☐ Is willing to serve as a preceptor. Consistently contributes to the team effort by assisting peers and members of the healthcare team May mentor others in providing care.	☐ Is willing to serve as a preceptor. Always contributes to the team effort by assisting peers and members of the healthcare team Acts as a mentor and resource for other nurses.
Communicate Effectively	☐ Is willing to share knowledge with new staff. Exhibits basic clinical judgment in nursing practice. Utilizes effective communication skills with peers and members of healthcare team. Needs prompting or direction on what to communication to Manger and care team to provide for safe learning environment. Demonstrates profession behavior, but may need assistance with conflict resolution. May need assistance with offering constructive feedback.	☐ Some experience with sharing knowledge with staff. Possesses increased clinical judgment and can apply knowledge into practice. Models empathetic and effective communication with peers and members of healthcare team. Needs minimal assistance in communication with Manager are care team to provide for safe learning environment. Demonstrates professional behavior and is able to seek appropriate resolution in difficult and/or conflicting circumstances. May need minimal assistance with offering constructive feedback	☐ Acts as a clinical resource for staff. Excellent clinical judgment and anticipation of needs in practice. Models exceptional communication abilities in routine practice and in critical events. Independent in communication to manager and team to provide for a safe learning environment Presents professional behavior in daily practice and is skilled at conflict resolution. He/she is a motivator and demonstrates team leadership through the appropriate offering of constructive feedback.
Recognize & Develop Others	☐ Demonstrates clinical judgment by explaining the "why" of decisions Excitement for learning and maintains intellectual curiosity Is able to work with varying styles of learning, incorporates learning curves, and learning timeframes into the preceptee's experiences with some guidance.	Demonstrates solid clinical judgment with explanations of decisions. Maintains excitement for learning and passion for teaching. Embraces varying styles of learning, incorporates learning curves, and learning timeframes independently into the preceptee's experiences Some experience with precepting.	☐ Exceptional clinical judgment with decisions Maintains a significant passion for Nursing and teaching. Role models the acceptance of varying styles of learning, learning curves, and learning timeframes into the preceptee's experiences. Skilled preceptor
Criteria	Competent level Column #1	Proficient level Column #2	Expert level Column #3
Add number of boxes checked in each column, then multiply by the column number			
Example: column #1 has 1 boxes checked, column #2 has 2, column #3 has 2	_____ X 1 = _____	_____ X 2 = _____	_____ X 3 = _____
1x1 = 1 2x2 = 4 3x2 = 6 11	Column 1 + Column 2 + Column 3 = Point Total _____ + _____ + _____ = _____		
Point Totals	Competent: 5-9	Proficient: 10-14	Expert: 15

This tool provides guidance for necessary growth required to meet the next preceptor level.

Preceptor Candidate Signature _____ Date _____

Preceptor Candidate Name (printed) _____

Manager Signature _____ Date _____

Manager Name (printed) _____

This form in its entirety, including your manager's signature, is required to gain entrance into the Preceptor Workshop.

Figure 12.3 Legacy Health Nursing Preceptor Rubric
Source: Legacy Health. Copyrighted. Used with permission.

The rubric format also serves as an objective classification of nurses' precepting experience. For managers, the nursing preceptor rubric provides formulaic evaluation criteria for the preceptors and detailed selection guidelines for matching preceptors with preceptees. For preceptors, the nursing preceptor rubric provides a clear evaluation of their precepting performance levels. Formalizing an integrated classification tool promotes consistent feedback, provides opportunities for coaching, and encourages transparent communication between the nurse manager and the preceptor. The development of preceptors following an integrated classification tool provides guidelines to construct an action plan to coach preceptors' growth process. Establishing organizational core performance standards and utilizing an integrated classification tool provide the nurse manager with a framework for a simple and repeatable preceptor selection process.

Setting the Stage

Matching preceptors and preceptees begins before new employees are interviewed or nurses are identified to expand their skills. The manager must understand the current needs of the organization and the specific unit/department. Bringing a new employee into a unit/department needs a well thought-out plan. The nurses must work together as a team to accomplish the many goals and tasks assigned to them on a daily basis. Onboarding new team members must be a decision that the majority of staff values and supports. The next step is to determine the specific needs of the unit/department: Are there enough resources to allow a new graduate nurse to develop? Is the unit better able to transition a nurse into a specialty environment? Do you lack clinical experience or staff who have specific knowledge and clinical skills needed in your unit? Is it time to advance the skills of one of your current nurses? After the nurse manager has determined the type of candidate needed, the process of matching a preceptor and preceptee should begin.

Interviewing potential employees is a wonderful opportunity to obtain some insight into candidates' personalities, learning styles, and feedback preferences. During the interview, it is helpful to ask questions that specifically address these areas. The interview process is an opportunity to better understand what type of preceptor the potential employee needs. Think about the unique personality traits, teaching styles, and feedback methods that your identified preceptors have that might lend them to forming a better bond with your new hire.

The manager should share with potential candidates (preceptees) the requirements needed to successfully complete the onboarding process or advancement of their clinical/

leadership skills and provide a brief overview of what the unit can offer as far as orientation, onboarding, preceptorship, mentorship, and educational opportunities. Be sure to share that candidates/preceptees are expected to be active participants in the process who should communicate if they do not feel things are going well. Candidates need to know that the organization and unit/department support additional team members. The unit's goal is to make new team members highly successful.

As the nurse manager, you understand how time-consuming the onboarding process is. You need to communicate the time commitment and expectations during the orientation phase. Individual motivation is essential to successful integration into a new team. Look for this commitment during the interview process.

As part of the decision to make an offer to potential candidates or to give advanced clinical opportunities to existing staff members, consider the best preceptor match for individuals. This ensures the preceptor resources are available to support your decision. Approach this decision in a proactive manner.

Your preceptors need to have strong communication skills and they need to be coached in giving constructive feedback to their preceptees. Feedback from colleagues or preceptors feels less punitive than when someone in line authority (for example, the manager) addresses the same issue, although ultimately it is the manager's job to ensure that feedback is given. Coaching by the manager can develop the preceptor's ability to address issues in the moment in a thoughtful and professional manner.

Conflict Considerations

What happens when a wonderful preceptor and a preceptee do not make a good match? The nurse manager must intervene in a supportive, nonjudgmental manner to understand immediately why the match is not working. Personality characteristics, learning styles, communication methods, individual expectations, education level, and individual behavior are all potential problem areas. Deciphering if the mismatch is a clinical or behavioral issue will determine how to proceed.

For learning style and teaching style mismatches, the manager must share this diagnosis and support the pair. The manager should act as a coach to develop an action plan with the preceptor and preceptee to bridge the gap. Preceptees must understand their personal learning styles so that their preceptors can guide learning activities to help them achieve success (Brunt & Kopp, 2007). Regular meetings with the preceptee and preceptor, both individually and together, are imperative to ensure that goals are being met. Proactively addressing issues can lead to enhanced retention and reduced time in orientation/onboarding (Brunt & Kopp, 2007).

If the divide between a preceptor and preceptee is too wide, you might need to change the preceptor. If the preceptee or preceptor identifies a mismatch, the person who brought the information forward should be praised for honestly sharing his or her discomfort or unmet needs. If this is a true mismatch, talking with each party individually and assigning a new preceptor whose personality and teaching style are a better fit usually puts things back on track.

Even the most thoughtful pairing might not work. If the mismatch stems from behavioral issues, the manager and preceptor need to institute an action plan for the preceptee. It is much easier for the preceptee and the entire team to address concerns early on. The preceptee must be coached on expectations and consequences. The manager must follow through on continued concerns to ensure that solutions are in place before the new hire becomes a permanent member of the team.

It is the manager's role to ensure adequate resources are available for the preceptor and preceptee pairing to be successful. The nurse manager is responsible for allocating time to the preceptor and preceptee to address goals and evaluate that clinical assignments are appropriate based on the needs and skill level of the preceptee. Each preceptor and preceptee comes to the table with varied strengths and skill levels. It is the nurse manager's responsibility to develop those strengths and skills to their highest potential. This fosters an engaged and sustainable workforce.

Preceptor Education

The preceptor is the nurse who forms the profession of nursing, one nurse at a time. The manager must recognize the value in initial and ongoing formal preceptor education. A strong clinician is not always a solid preceptor. Workshops specifically tailored to the preceptor role should be formally established and regularly offered. Concepts offered in preceptor workshops—adult learning theory, communication, socialization, and clinical judgment—need to be part of a continual learning process for all preceptors. The sustained future of nursing depends upon the aptitude of preceptors. This requires initial and ongoing education to promote preceptor proficiency.

Communication

Maintaining open and honest communication for a safe environment begins with leaders listening to those closest to the issues. A manager's active participation and consistent facilitation of regular communication among preceptor, manager, and preceptee promote successful employees. To ensure adequate support for new employees, nurse managers should set formal meetings, implement impromptu check-ins, establish open office hours, and frequently review documentation. A framework for establishing formal meetings with preceptors and preceptees—with suggested time frames, areas of focus, and follow-up—is provided in Table 12.2.

Table 12.2	**Suggested Guidelines for Formal Meetings**		
Time frame	*Meeting participants*	*Focus*	*Next Steps*
Initial: After 3-5 shifts	Manager, preceptee, preceptor	• Establish preceptor/ preceptee relationship • Set initial goals; plan for competency progression • Review self-assessment • Review set orientation documentation • Provide opportunities for feedback	Set timeline for next meeting
Midway: Halfway through planned onboarding/ orientation timeline	Manager, preceptee, preceptor	• Discuss how far new employee progressed and where next focus is • Discuss transition of preceptors • Provide opportunities for feedback • Review set orientation documentation	Set timeline for next meeting

Table 12.2 Suggested Guidelines for Formal Meetings (cont.)			
Near end: 2 weeks prior to end of onboarding/ orientation timeline	Manager, preceptee, preceptor	• Discuss what still needs to be accomplished for successful orientation • Review set onboarding/ orientation documentation • Provide opportunities for feedback	Set timeline for onboarding/ orientation completion
Additional: Scheduled as needed	Manager, preceptee, preceptor	• What has been accomplished so far, and what needs to be current focus • Provide opportunities for feedback • Review set onboarding/ orientation documentation	Recognition of accomplishment

Managers can also use organizational opportunities to support their preceptors. Newsletters are an excellent form of communication. A newsletter can provide a venue for supporting and recognizing that the institution values the preceptor role. Dissemination of information can be a means of supporting preceptor education.

Preceptor forums are an excellent format to get feedback and input into the ongoing development and modification of the preceptor program. Insights into the preceptors' work are invaluable in creating an environment that supports networking, creative problem solving, and unity of purpose. Barriers to a successful clinical preceptor program are often best resolved by the nurses providing direct patient care, preceptors, and preceptees.

Guidance

The manager role is critical in establishing a successful preceptor program. The key components of a successful program include an atmosphere of trust between preceptors, collaborative goals for demonstrating competencies, and support for learning experiences. The preceptor and preceptee pair needs time set aside for reflection or debriefing. All components are dependent upon communication among preceptors, preceptees, the manager, and other stakeholders, such as charge nurses. Establishing a preceptorship that is conducive to teachable moments is crucial. The manager should be focused on providing an environment of learning, which includes appropriate assignments, exposure to learning opportunities, time for review of standards, evaluation of goals, and time for debriefing. Make assignments in regard to the preceptee's learning needs. The preceptor and preceptee should not "divide and conquer" to complete the tasks of the assignment in a timely manner. They need to work side-by-side to ensure that the preceptor is there when teachable moments arise. In the clinical setting, teachable moments are missed if the preceptor and preceptee are in different patient rooms when care is being provided.

Preceptor Evaluation

Managers play a key role in the evaluation process for their preceptors. Evaluating preceptors based on the organizational core performance standards is important for improving the preceptor process. Seeking out all relevant sources of feedback and filtering them into the final evaluation are the first responsibilities of the manager in the evaluation process. Coordination of evaluations from preceptees, educators, charge nurses, peers, and other stakeholders should be part of a preceptor evaluation. Incorporating peer feedback is crucial for preceptor growth, because that feedback is often the most relevant in content and honest in context. Focusing peer feedback on organization, prioritization, clinical judgment, communication, use of resources, and teamwork enables a broad evaluation of the preceptor's practice. A sample preceptor evaluation is shown in Figure 12.4. Utilizing a standardized form for your evaluations supports consistency. Reviewing and updating the evaluation form depending upon unit needs and preceptor and preceptee feedback can ensure continual improvement.

Managers should schedule meeting time with their preceptors to discuss the evaluation. Preceptor feedback has the greatest impact during or immediately after the precepting process. Yearly staff evaluations and end of orientation evaluations for the new hire are existing processes that can also address preceptor performance. Managers must make preceptor evaluations a priority to grow and support their nurse preceptors.

The manager's primary role with preceptor evaluation is to provide coaching. Having formalized organizational core performance standards assists managers in this process. Individual preceptor performance must mirror these set standards. Evaluation should be supportive and aimed at growth, and managers should plan with their preceptors how this growth can occur. This collaborative effort can help ensure necessary support for your preceptors and new hires.

LEGACY
HEALTH

Preceptor Evaluation

Evaluation of: _____ By_____

Date: _____

Competency Level Key: 1=Never, 2= Rarely, 3=Sometimes, 4=Very Often 5=Always

Organization	Level	Comments
1. Supports/teaches organizational process		
2. Promotes delegation		
3. Able to adjust precepting to changing situations		
4. Adapts teaching style to meet preceptee's needs		
5. Individualizes precepting process		
Prioritizing	**Level**	**Comments**
1. Helps preceptee develop their plan of care		
2. Develops understanding of care priorities		
Clinical Judgment	**Level**	**Comments**
1. Helps develop clinical judgment process		
2. Supports anticipation of care needs and interventions		
3. Provided reasonable explanations or rationale for nursing actions		
4. Promotes learning by asking open-ended questions		
Communication	**Level**	**Comments**
1. Provides routine feedback		
2. Interacts with others in a professional manner		
3. Provides positive learning environment		
4. Open and amicable to feedback		
Use of Resources	**Level**	**Comments**
1. Follows policy and procedures correctly		
2. Consistently productive		
3. Shows preceptee the available resources		
Team Work	**Level**	**Comments**
1. Encourages team work		
2. Supportive of preceptee		
3. Provided adequate support for preceptee		

Things to address/Other Comments: _____
_____
_____

Figure 12.4   Legacy Health Preceptor Evaluation

Source: Legacy Health. Copyrighted. Used with permission.

Eliciting preceptor and preceptee feedback regarding their perceptions of the entire orientation program can drive process improvement. Meeting expectations, praising positive outcomes, and planning for how to deal with unexpected situations are topics for discussion. In practice, this feedback often surfaces during a crisis. Being proactive in discussing any problems before they arise provides the most support for your preceptors and preceptees.

A transparent and consistent approach is essential for preceptors to understand and be accountable for their role performance. Such an approach enables preceptors to alter their practice to meet the set standard. Managers can then hold preceptors accountable for the selection criteria or use the standards to set performance goals. Follow-through is essential.

After the selection criteria are in place, manager support for the process is essential for preceptor program success. As Studer (2009) states, "Remember, what we permit, we promote. What we allow, we encourage. . . . It's better not to have a standard in place than to have it and not hold people accountable for it; it looks insincere and makes employees think other standards can be ignored, too" (p. 135). Manager accountability to the process is essential for the rest of the team to follow.

Recognition of Preceptors

Preceptors play a crucial role in the success and development of staff. Their guidance and support of new employees or current nurses who are advancing their skills are fundamental in nursing. Preceptors are responsible not only for ensuring that preceptees are competent, but also for continually role-modeling professional behavior. With such an important role, how do the manager and the organization ensure that preceptors have recognition for the valuable role they play?

Meaningful recognition comes in many forms. It is personal, and it can often be difficult for those receiving recognition to articulate what truly makes them feel recognized. Recognition is not always a grand, sweeping gesture, and what makes your preceptors feel recognized might vary immensely from nurse to nurse.

Asking a nurse to consider becoming a preceptor can be a morale boost in itself. This past year, our organization used a form of Benner's novice to expert model to create a model for precepting (Benner, 1984). In the past, we relied heavily on expert nurses to precept our new employees and new nurse graduates. When we utilized our newer, "competent" nurses, those nurses felt recognized and valued. These new preceptors demonstrated a sense of confidence and pride in their new role.

After the manager and unit staff acknowledge a colleague as a preceptor, they have many ways available to provide meaningful recognition. Some examples are shown in Table 12.3. The preceptor's effort, energy, and guidance toward the professional development of fellow staff can be recognized via professional, financial, or personal means. Clinical ladders can be a means to advance nursing practice, and recognition could come in the form of higher pay or professional advancement. Preceptor pay differentials provide financial incentives and recognition. Organizations without embedded financial incentives for preceptors can still provide meaningful recognition by eliminating the preceptors from forced cancellation rotations while they are precepting, or they can be given preference when applying to attend conferences or special educational opportunities.

Meaningful recognition for preceptors can come in the form of official praise by nominating them for awards within the organization, unit, and local and national professional organizations. Managers can continue to foster preceptors' leadership and development by requesting their assistance on system-wide committees and projects. At the unit level, managers can have preceptees nominate their preceptors for recognition and then announce the winners during staff meetings or in unit newsletters.

Still, the most meaningful recognition might come in the form of a simple "thank you"— acknowledging the important role preceptors play in the cohesiveness and success of the organization and unit. Recognizing their efforts and including them as part of the reason the preceptees are successful can fill preceptors with a sense of pride and accomplishment.

Table 12.3   Example of Preceptor Recognition
• Clinical ladder advancement
• Preceptor differential
• No forced cancellation rotations
• Paid conference or educational day
• Authoring newsletter articles for preceptors
• Preceptor of the year award
• Highlight and post individual preceptor biographies
• Special thank-you at staff meetings
• Preceptor pin or pen

Getting Creative to Overcome Challenges

A manager is not an island; managers need to remember that they work with a team of highly skilled clinicians and leaders. Successful managers use members of their teams to help ensure creative solutions for tackling limited orientation and onboarding hours, heavy assignments, budgetary constraints, and overall lack of time. Unit-based roles such as chairs of preceptor or mentorship councils, charge nurses, supervisors, and unit educators can assist the manager in establishing and implementing the onboarding/orientation process. These unit-based leaders are instrumental in the success of any precepting program. By utilizing a shared governance model, managers can reach out to members of their teams to support both the preceptor and preceptee. The more team members are involved in the functioning of the unit, the more likely they are to be engaged and vested in the success of all team members.

A mentorship program can help extend the support offered to a new employee. For example, a unit-based mentorship council that pairs a new employee with a mentor for a time period (3-6 months post orientation) can provide extended clinical and socialization support. The mentor should not be one of the new employee's original preceptors. Utilizing other staff to assist in the mentorship process expands the new employee's network of support. The chair of the mentorship council and the unit manager can monitor the mentorship program. They can establish frequent meetings and use formalized feedback tools to help identify further learning opportunities and areas of further development, or assist in support by recognizing accomplishments. A mentorship program might enable a team to extend clinical support to the new employee without extending the onboarding/orientation budget. This clinical mentorship model can also be successful in helping existing staff who are struggling with clinical issues or who need support with skill advancement.

Finding time for preceptors and preceptees to evaluate their shift, discuss new concepts, or elaborate on teachable moments can be a challenge. Some potential strategies for the preceptor are shown in Table 12.4. The unit charge nurses can play an important role in helping to provide time away from the bedside for the preceptor and preceptee to debrief. The unit charge nurses are tuned into the flow of the unit. They can identify periods where other staff members might have time to cover the preceptor's and preceptee's assignments to give them some time to meet.

Managers can coach staff on time management strategies to assist with preceptor feedback and communication. Often, if feedback is left to the end of the shift, it might not occur without entering into overtime pay. Individuals might be able to alter their workflow to provide the majority of the feedback during their clinical shift so that the end of the day debriefing can quickly occur.

Table 12.4 Time Management for Preceptors
• Work with your charge nurse to find uninterrupted time to review standards with your preceptee.
• Alter work flow to allow time to debrief with preceptee during the shift.
• Advocate for a patient assignment that promotes time for teaching.
• Choose assignments that focus on the preceptee's specific learning needs.
• Communicate needs.
• Collaborate with your manager to complete orientation and competency requirements.

Conclusion

Investing in the development of your unit by fostering staff to become preceptors and by successfully growing new staff is one of the greatest legacies you can offer to your profession and your organization. By creating a strong and successful unit that supports, recognizes, and embraces new nurses, you will have advanced the profession of nursing by ensuring high quality outcomes for the patients and families who are entrusted in your care.

References

American Nurses Association (ANA). (2001). *Code of ethics for nurses with interpretive statements*. Silver Spring, MD: Author.

American Nurses Association (ANA). (2010). *Nursing: Scope and standards of practice* (2nd ed.). Silver Spring, MD: Author.

Beecroft, P., Hernandez, A. M., & Reid, D. (2008). Team preceptorships: A new approach for precepting new nurses. *Journal for Nurses in Staff Development, 24*(4), 143-148.

Benner, P. (1984). *From novice to expert: Excellence and power in clinical nursing practice*. Menlo Park, CA: Addison-Wesley Publishing Company.

Brunt, B. A., & Kopp, D. J. (2007). Impact of preceptor and orientee learning styles on satisfaction: A pilot study. *Journal for Nurses in Staff Development, 23*(1), 36-44.

Myrick, F., & Yonge, O. (2005). *Nursing preceptorship: Connecting practice & education*. Philadelphia, PA: Lippincott Williams & Wilkins.

Studer, Q. (2009). *Straight A leadership: Alignment, action, accountability*. Gulf Breeze, FL: Fire Starter Publishing.

Preceptor Development Plan **For Managers: Selecting, Supporting, and Sustaining Preceptors**			

Review the information on selecting, supporting, and sustaining preceptors described in this chapter. What are your strengths? In which areas do you need to increase your knowledge and expertise? What is your plan for expanding your knowledge and expertise? What resources are available? Who can help you?

Review your organization's preceptor performance standards, selection criteria, education program (initial and continuing), evaluation forms, and recognition plans. If any of these are not yet available in your organization, work with stakeholders to develop and implement them.

Name:			
Establishing Preceptor Performance Standards			
Strengths	Needs	Plan	Resources
Preceptor Selection Criteria			
Strengths	Needs	Plan	Resources
Matching Preceptors and Preceptees			
Strengths	Needs	Plan	Resources
Conflict Considerations			
Strengths	Needs	Plan	Resources
Preceptor Education			
Strengths	Needs	Plan	Resources
Preceptor Evaluations			
Strengths	Needs	Plan	Resources
Preceptor Recognition			
Strengths	Needs	Plan	Resources
Overcoming Challenges			
Strengths	Needs	Plan	Resources

Note: This form and other resources are available at www.RNPreceptor.com.

"That no man can sincerely try to help another without helping himself . . . it is one of the most beautiful compensations in life."

–Ralph Waldo Emerson

The Practice of Self-Care to Prevent Burnout and Create the Optimal Healing Environment

13

Kim Richards, RN

OBJECTIVES

- Understand the importance of self-care for yourself and others

- Develop an individualized plan of self-care practices for yourself

The calling to the nursing profession is a powerful pull, full of heartfelt compassion, deep care for others, and a strong desire to make a difference in the lives of others. The need to consistently "give" requires courage, resiliency, and mandatory refilling of personal reservoirs. Nurses cannot continue to give from an empty basket. Soul-nurturing, life-affirming activities that renew energy, compassion, and engagement in the profession are as important to learn and practice as any other requirement of a professional nurse's life. Preceptors, who are assuming the responsibility for teaching others in addition to maintaining their own knowledge and expertise, need to pay particular attention to self-care. They also have the opportunity, as part of precepting, to teach others to make self-care a priority.

This chapter discusses self-care, compassion fatigue, and their relationship; pathways to promote self-care practices; the benefits of making self-care a priority in one's own life, debunking the myth that self-care is "self-ish"; and practical suggestions applicable for a nurse's busy lifestyle. Sustainable self-care practices do not always require large amounts of time but can be moments of mindful activities strung together throughout the day, creating respite from stressors, from feeling overwhelmed, and from ending up mentally, physically, and emotionally exhausted.

What is self-care? Cheryl Richardson (2009), long considered the guru of self-care, simply states, "Self-care is extraordinary mothering of self in mind, body and spirit" (p. 12). A recent study ($N = 20$ care units) identified that self-care had a significant relationship with teamwork with nurses ($r = .519$, $p < .019$; Hozak & Brennan, 2011). Another study of staff nurses ($N = 65$) revealed self-care has a negative relationship with both compassion fatigue ($r = -.61$, $p < .001$) and burnout ($r = -.61$, $p < .001$; Johnson, 2011).

Compassion fatigue is a physical and emotional exhaustion that causes a decline in a person's ability to feel compassion when taking care of others. It is the cumulative result of internalizing the emotions of patients, coworkers, family, and friends. It costs the health care industry millions of dollars each year in stress, burnout, and employee turnover. Compassion fatigue is a result of the caregiver being focused on providing care to others and *not* providing care to themselves. Providing care cannot be a one-way street, especially for health care professionals. Too often, health care professionals give most of themselves to others over a long period of time and don't stop to recharge their own batteries (Richards, 2011).

Dr. Barbara Dossey, founder of the Theory of Integral Nursing, has identified six key elements, or pathways, of self-care (Dossey & Keegan, 2008). The pathways are physical, mental, emotional, spiritual, relationships, and choices. You will notice that some of the same self-care suggestions are repeated in several pathways. That is because some action steps have a global effect on self-care.

Physical

Your physical health is your responsibility and yours alone. To practice self-care and healthy living, education and knowledge are essential to determining what is best for you. Your body is the only vehicle carrying you from birth to death, so routine maintenance is a no-brainer! Listen to your body, take charge, and tune in to changes and sensations. Be keenly aware of the undeniable connection between your mind and your body, as the dynamic is constant. As you strengthen your body, you will experience a mirrored effect in all areas of your life. Physical pathway suggestions are shown in Table 13.1.

Table 13.1   Physical Pathway Suggestions

- Get an exercise buddy.
- Drinks lots of water (at least eight glasses per day) and take a multivitamin.
- Take deep, slow breaths often throughout the day.
- Plan ahead for quick, healthy meals.
- Take a walk outside.
- Intentionally touch one person a day.
- Meditate or set aside alone-time for 10 minutes a day.
- Schedule all preventive health appointments.
- Schedule a massage/facial/manicure/pedicure on a routine basis.
- Pet my dog or cat.
- De-clutter my bedroom to create a restful, calm environment for sleep.
- Go to bed an hour early once a week and read.
- Avoid TV before bed or in bed.
- Soak in a warm bath.
- Forgive myself or others. Release emotional baggage.
- Take a laugh break! Daily comics, funny people, humorous situations . . . just laugh!
- Exercise at least three times per week.
- Always eat breakfast.
- When planning meetings with food, order healthy choices.
- Keep a notepad by my bed to write down and release worries for later. Take time to rest.
- Keep healthy snacks nearby and restock often.
- Put cloth over my computer when done to signify "work done."
- Take a 15-minute nap.
- Know my BMI and keep it 25 or lower.
- Create a sanctuary at work and at home.
- Schedule a play date or game night.

Mental

Flexibility, open mindedness, and constant learning are the pillars of a healthy mental environment. Our brains possess unlimited, mostly untapped potential; but, similar to our muscles, some "heavy lifting" is required to grow and blossom. As self-care applications are practiced, you might find your brain seems to relax, focus, and retain more than ever.

This concept gives new meaning to the adage "food for thought." You might find yourself becoming more mindful of how your environment feeds your brain. Mental pathway suggestions are found in Table 13.2.

Table 13.2   Mental Pathway Suggestions
• Ask for help *before* I feel overwhelmed. Make a "how you can support me" list.
• Create a sanctuary at work and at home.
• Stop watching mindless TV or negative news media, especially before bed.
• Take deep, slow breaths and close my eyes periodically throughout the day.
• Create a "vision board" of how I want my life to be.
• Start the day with a positive affirmation, and then expect a good day.
• Create a wall or collage of mementos that trigger appreciation, gratitude, and joy.
• Take a walk and connect with nature by spending time outside.
• Meditate or set aside alone-time for 10 minutes a day.
• Eliminate any appointments that are not necessary.
• Weed my garden of friends. Keep only those where friendship is a two-way street.
• Create a success team to reach my goals.
• Pet my dog or cat.
• Have a "safe" friend or colleague to talk with or vent to.
• Forgive myself and others. Release emotional baggage.
• Listen to inspirational music on the way to work, during breaks at work, and on the way home.
• Take a laugh break! Daily comics, funny people, humorous situations . . . just laugh!
• Exercise at least three times per week.
• Light a candle and set the tone for relaxation and positive moods.
• Consider hiring a crew for cleaning or outdoor chores once a month. My time is valuable. How much am I worth?
• Read a book and discuss with others.
• Take public transportation to ease the stress of traffic.
• Refuse to listen to a rumor or nasty gossip. Speak up.
• Keep a notepad by my bed to write down and release worries for later. Take time to rest.
• Say "no" without feeling guilty once a day.
• Put cloth over my computer when done to signify "work done."

- When walking out of work, physically "throw away" worries in the trash can. Reverse the action on the way into work by "throwing away" worries from home.
- De-clutter my closet and bedroom. Donate unused items and clothes. Create my bedroom for calmness and sleeping, not working.
- Never allow computers or cell phones in bed.
- Know that by taking action first, the feeling will follow.
- Create a support network.
- Distance myself from too many people leaning heavily on me at once.
- Take a 15-minute nap.
- Talk kindly to my reflection in the mirror. Pump it up!
- Buy a bunch of flowers.
- Reward myself for milestones or accomplishments.

Emotional

Emotions are a dominant part of the human condition. We engage in constant dialogue within ourselves; how we feel, perceive, and respond is regulated by our emotional state. Past joys, hurts, and traumatic experiences all contribute to our emotional health, yet we also can choose to release toxic feelings that cause us to be repeatedly victimized. Identifying where unresolved emotion is eroding your self-care is freeing for both you and those around you. Emotional pathway suggestions are found in Table 13.3.

Table 13.3   Emotional Pathway Suggestions

- Find a photo that reminds me of a happy childhood memory.
- Stop watching mindless TV or negative news media, especially before bed.
- Collect items or pictures that reignite and reflect my spirit.
- Journal daily about how I feel.
- Start the day with a positive affirmation and expect a good day.
- Create a wall or collage of mementos that trigger appreciation, gratitude, and joy.
- Take a walk.
- Connect with nature by spending time outside.
- Weed my garden of friends. Keep only those where friendship is a two-way street.
- Take 10 minutes of alone-time per day.
- Pet my dog or cat.

Table 13.3   Emotional Pathway Suggestions (cont.)

- Have a "safe" friend or colleague to talk with or vent to.
- Forgive myself and others. Release emotional baggage.
- Listen to inspirational music on the way to work, during breaks at work, and on the way home.
- Take a laugh break! Daily comics, funny people, humorous situations . . . just laugh!
- Exercise at least three times per week.
- Light a candle and set the tone for relaxation and positive moods.
- Consider hiring a crew for cleaning or outdoor chores once a month. My time is valuable. How much am I worth?
- Read books and discuss with others.
- Take time to talk with children or grandchildren.
- Take public transportation to ease the stress of traffic.
- Refuse to listen to a rumor or nasty gossip. Speak up.
- Say "no" without feeling guilty once a day.
- Put a cloth over my computer when done to signify "work done."
- When walking out of work, physically "throw away" worries in trash can. Reverse the action on the way into work by "throwing away" worries from home.
- De-clutter my closet and bedroom. Donate unused items and clothes.
- Create my bedroom for calmness and sleeping, not working.
- Never allow computers or cell phones in bed.
- Know that by taking action first, the feeling will follow.
- Create a support network.
- Distance myself from too many people leaning heavily on me at once.
- Encourage others in their self-care practices.
- Talk kindly to my reflection in the mirror. Pump it up!
- Buy myself flowers.
- Reward myself for milestones or accomplishments.
- Keep a notepad by my bed to write down and release worries for later. Take time to rest.
- Create a sanctuary at work and at home.
- Find an old friend and reconnect.
- Say "I love you" three times per day.
- Support or donate to a cause of my choice.
- Mentor someone. Pass on my blessings.

Spiritual

Spiritual self-care is a reflection of your belief, in a very personal way, in a higher power than yourself that connects you with the universe. Your beliefs might or might not be deeply rooted in organized religious practices, rituals, or celebrations, but the spirit that you reflect is unique to you. Your beliefs shape your perceptions of your world; therefore, they serve to nurture your soul or deplete your spirit. Spiritual pathway suggestions are found in Table 13.4.

Table 13.4   Spiritual Pathway Suggestions
• Express my servant leadership purpose by being an example of "flow."
• Collect items or pictures that reignite or reflect my spirit.
• Connect with nature by spending time outside.
• Journal about comments, situations, or people who reconnect me to my "calling." Tell others.
• Allow myself to receive compassion before giving it away.
• Meditate for 10 minutes a day.
• Light a candle and ask for guidance.
• Create a vision board of my legacy.
• Create a support network. Join a like-minded study group.
• Encourage others in their self-care practices.
• Create a sanctuary at work and at home.
• Volunteer my time and talent to a cause important to me.
• Attend spiritual services or celebrations.
• Spend 5 minutes stargazing.
• Reconnect with my spiritual beliefs.
• Support or donate to a cause of my choice.
• Find a photo that reminds me of a happy childhood memory.
• Ask a colleague to compliment me on three attributes that contribute to my life purpose.
• Take 10 minutes of alone-time per day.

Relationships

Your life is dynamic. The quality of relationships in which you participate is a direct reflection of how you see yourself. Increasing awareness of the impact of relationships that either add to or subtract from your life can be a lifelong process. This element of self-care can be illusive and requires identification of cohesiveness or disharmony. Your relationship with yourself is the foundation from which all others flow. Relationship pathway suggestions are shown in Table 13.5.

Table 13.5   Relationships Pathway Suggestions
• Write a note to someone I care for.
• Collect items or pictures that reignite and reflect my spirit.
• Create a wall or collage of mementos that triggers appreciation, gratitude, and joy.
• Intentionally touch one person each day.
• Weed my garden of friends. Keep only those where friendship is a two-way street.
• Create a success team to reach my goals.
• Pet my dog or cat.
• Have a "safe" friend or colleague to talk with or vent to.
• Forgive myself and others. Release emotional baggage.
• Read a book and discuss with others.
• Take time to talk with children or grandchildren.
• Refuse to listen to a rumor or nasty gossip. Speak up.
• When walking out of work, physically "throw away" worries in trash can. Reverse the action on the way into work by "throwing away" worries from home.
• Create my bedroom for calmness and sleeping, not working.
• Never allow computers or cell phones in bed.
• Create a support network. Encourage others in their self-care practices.
• Find an old friend and reconnect.
• Say "I love you" at least three times per day.
• Compliment two coworkers today.
• Volunteer my time and talent to an important cause.
• Mentor a child.
• Schedule a play date or game night.
• Support or donate to a cause of my choice.
• Ask a colleague to compliment me on three attributes.

Choices

Your life is precisely where it is currently because of the choices you have made, both those labeled "good" and those "not so good." When you make choices from a place of self-compassion and the choices are in line with your core values, neither self-sacrifice nor self-flagellation has a place. Your journey to improved self-care and harmony within can be naturally enhanced by your heightened awareness of your values, desires, and what makes your heart sing. When you choose to fully participate in your own life, listening to your authentic spirit and giving yourself permission to take action, you begin to fly! Choices pathway suggestions are found in Table 13.6.

Table 13.6   Choices Pathway Suggestions

- Plan ahead for quick, healthy meals.
- Take a walk.
- Intentionally touch one person each day.
- Meditate for 10 minutes a day.
- Eliminate any appointments that are not necessary.
- Weed my garden of friends. Keep only those where friendship is a two-way street.
- Create a success team to reach my goals.
- Schedule all preventive health appointments.
- Take 10 minutes of alone-time per day.
- Have a "safe" friend or colleague to talk with or vent to.
- Forgive myself and others. Release emotional baggage.
- Listen to inspirational music on the way to work, during breaks at work, and on the way home.
- Take a laugh break! Daily comics, funny people, humorous situations . . . just laugh!
- Exercise at least three times per week.
- Consider hiring a crew for cleaning or outdoor chores once a month. My time is valuable. How much am I worth?
- Read a book and discuss with others.
- Take time to talk with children or grandchildren.
- Take public transportation to ease the stress of traffic.
- Always eat breakfast. When planning meetings with food, order healthy choices.
- Refuse to listen to a rumor or nasty gossip. Speak up.
- Keep healthy snacks nearby and restock often.
- Say "no" without feeling guilty, once a day.

Table 13.6   Choices Pathway Suggestions (cont.)

- When walking out of work, physically "throw away" worries in trash can. Reverse the action on the way into work by "throwing away" worries from home.
- Distance myself from too many people leaning heavily on me at once.
- Create a support network.
- Take a 15-minute nap.
- Know that by taking action first, the feeling will follow.
- Reward myself for milestones or accomplishments.

Conclusion

Connecting with your strengths and the values they represent is what energizes you! Your strengths make you feel more alive and reflect your life passions. The pathways to self-care have no hierarchy; each affects the other. They are interconnected and often work in tandem to create self-compassion, self-awareness, and life harmony. When you identify and incorporate them more fully into your life, your overall life satisfaction improves. Using your strengths to cultivate areas you choose to enhance can allow you to develop a more balanced self-care journey and overall capacity for resilience. Developing each pathway more fully might require self-compassion and identification of a void. Addition of self-care practices that support these new insights requires a balance of skill and challenge. The most critical action is to keep moving forward, "trying on" what resonates with you and what seems to fit with your lifestyle. After some practice and commitment, you will find the steps you are taking becoming less uncomfortable and more routine; eventually the steps will be effortlessly habitual.

Developing self-nurturing habits and healthy coping skills and proactively practicing self-care daily are the first steps in creating a firm foundation for growth, productivity, and sustained engagement. Being mindful of triggers that can cause disharmony and confidently knowing your self-affirming routines allow you to rise above the immediate stressors and expand your capacity for resiliency.

References

Dossey, B., & Keegan, L. (2008). *Holistic nursing: A handbook for practice*. Sudbury, MA: Jones and Bartlett.

Hozak, M. A., & Brennan, M. (2012). Caring at the core: Maximizing the likelihood that a caring moment will occur. In J. Nelson & J. Watson (Eds.), *Measuring caring: International research in caritas as healing* (pp. 195-224). New York, NY: Springer Publishing Company, LLC.

Johnson, S. (2012). A U.S. study of nurses' self-care and compassion fatigue using Watson's concepts of caritas. In J. Nelson & J. Watson (Eds.), *Measuring caring: International research in caritas as healing* (pp. 413-420). New York, NY: Springer Publishing Company, LLC.

Richards, K. A. (2011, April 28). Self-Care Academy: My Self-Care Journey workshop.

Richardson, C. (2009). *The art of extreme self-care*. Carlsbad, CA: Hay House.

Preceptor Development Plan
The Practice of Self-Care to Prevent Burnout and Create an Optimal Healing Environment

Review the information on the practice of self-care to prevent burnout and create an optimal healing environment described in this chapter. Create a plan of self-care for yourself. To get started, pick three of the suggestions in each pathway and develop a plan on how to include those things in your life in the next month.

Name:	
Date:	
Physical Pathway Suggestions I Commit to Including in My Life This Month	
Suggestion	Plan
Mental Pathway Suggestions I Commit to Including in My Life This Month	
Suggestion	Plan
Emotional Pathway Suggestions I Commit to Including in My Life This Month	
Suggestion	Plan
Spiritual Pathway Suggestions I Commit to Including in My Life This Month	
Suggestion	Plan
Relationships Pathway Suggestions I Commit to Including in My Life This Month	
Suggestion	Plan
Choices Pathway Suggestions I Commit to Including in My Life This Month	
Suggestion	Plan

Note: This form and other resources are available at www.RNPreceptor.com.

Using *Mastering Precepting: A Nurse's Handbook for Success* for Preceptor Education

This book can be used as a resource for a preceptor education course. The following are suggestions for the use of each chapter.

Chapter 1: The Preceptor Role

- Review and discuss the ANA Standards of Practice and Professional Performance and the Code of Ethics and verify that everyone is familiar with the content. Ask participants for examples of standards from their specialty organizations.

- Discuss safety and quality as parts of the context of precepting.

- Discuss each preceptor role in general.

- If the organization has articulated values, review and discuss the values and how they can be integrated into precepting. Do the same for the nursing division. If the organization and/or the nursing division do not have their values articulated, divide the participants into small groups. Ask each group to come up with what they think the organization or division values, what it should value, and how these values can be integrated into precepting. Have each group present to the entire class and discuss the results.

- Divide the participants into groups and ask them to create a list of sacred cows and unwritten rules of the game in the organization and the nursing division. Have each group present to the entire class and discuss the results.

- Discuss lateral violence, disruptive behavior, and verbal abuse with the class. Ask for examples from the group and discuss strategies for preceptors to protect preceptees from such abuse.

Chapter 2: Learning: The Foundation of Precepting

- Review and discuss learning theories.

- Discuss role modeling. Ask the participants for recent examples of good and not-good role modeling that they have observed. Challenge them to compare what they do with their values. For example, if they value collaboration, ask for examples on how they collaborate with others.

- Discuss Maslow's hierarchy of needs and how preceptors can help preceptees move up the hierarchy.

- Ask participants to remember when they were a novice and describe how that felt. Discuss Benner's novice to expert model and how the model can be used in precepting. As a group, discuss strategies to support novices as they move toward expert practice.

- Discuss learning styles and engage participants in describing how they learn best.

- Ask participants to reflect on their own learning and experience. Ask: "What do you need to learn to be a competent, proficient, and then an expert preceptor? What experience do you have that will be applicable? What is your frame of reference? Are you ready to learn?"

- Ask participants: "Whom will you be precepting? Undergraduate nursing students? New graduate nurses? Experienced nurses entering a new specialty? How will you model for them what they need to learn?"

Chapter 3: Precepting Strategies

- Discuss the role expectations of preceptors in your organization.

- Discuss the model of precepting to be used in your organization (for example, single preceptee, cohorts). If more than one model is used, discuss all the models used and when each is used.

- If your organization has structured onboarding programs such as a new graduate residency or specialty preparation, discuss these programs and the preceptor role in them. Provide specific examples of how preceptors integrate in the programs and how communication about preceptees occurs between the programs and the preceptors.

- Discuss methods of communication between preceptors and other stakeholders (for example, the preceptee's manager, charge nurses). Ask the group to discuss facilitators and barriers to communication and strategies to promote facilitation and overcome barriers.

- Break into small groups and ask each group to come up with ground rules for preceptor-preceptee relationships. Discuss the results of the group work as a whole class.

- Discuss the transitions that preceptees go through and any support your organization has for such transitions (for example, career coach). If the organization does not have any support mechanisms in place, discuss what preceptors can do to support and engage others in supporting preceptee transitions.

- Discuss the strengths-based approach to clinical teaching.

- Break the group into pairs. Have one member of the pair be the preceptor and the other the preceptee. Have the preceptor do a 1-minute praising. Reverse roles and repeat. Bring the group back together and discuss the process.

- Review the microskills model. Use a case study to discuss the steps in the microskills model.

- Discuss debriefing. Ask the group for suggestions on how debriefing can be integrated into the busy day.

- Discuss reflective practice and ask for examples on how reflective practice can be used with preceptees.

- Discuss ending the preceptor-preceptee relationship. If your organization has a specific handoff procedure from the preceptor to the manager or an end-of-preceptorship summary form or status report, discuss how it is used. If these do not exist, talk as a group about how to best hand off the preceptee.

- Discuss any celebrations that your organization has to commemorate the preceptee completing the onboarding process. For example, many organizations with new graduate residencies have "graduation" or completion ceremonies to which hospital staff and preceptees' families are invited.

Chapter 4: Competence, Critical Thinking, Clinical Judgment and Reasoning, and Confidence

- Discuss what competence is.

- Review role competencies that your organization has adopted and how they are measured and validated. Review competency documentation systems.

- Discuss the Competency Outcomes and Performance Assessment model and its use in precepting.

- Discuss the core critical thinking skills.

- Using the key questions and a case study, have the group work through helping a preceptee learn how to think critically.

- Discuss clinical reasoning and the patterns of clinical reasoning that experienced nurses use. Use a case study in which clinical reasoning occurs, and ask the participants how to break down the reasoning steps for a novice nurse.

- Using Tanner's model of clinical judgment and a case study, ask participants to discuss how they would help a novice use clinical judgment.

- Ask participants to describe situations in which they used their intuition to act on a patient problem. Then ask them to identify the pattern or absence of a pattern that was occurring that was their cue to act.

- Discuss ways to promote confidence in preceptees.

Chapter 5: Having a Plan: Developing and Using Objectives, Goals, and Outcomes

- Discuss the concept of having a plan and the continuum of plans from a fully detailed written plan to taking a few minutes at the start of a shift to decide and discuss what the plan is for the patient and/or the day.

- Discuss what a goal is. Share the organization's and nursing division's goals as examples. Additional goals can also be shared, such as the goals of the new graduate residency.

- Compare objectives and outcomes.

- Have the participants create an example of a goal, outcome, and objectives.

- Review the taxonomies. Divide the participants into small groups and have participants create sample objectives in each knowledge dimension and domain, and at each level. Have some groups create examples of written objectives, some create examples of beginning of the shift objectives for working with one patient, and some create examples for the whole shift.

Chapter 6: Communication

- Discuss the five skills of effective communication: intent, listening, advocacy, inquiry, and silence.

- Practice using the questions for setting intent for the preceptor-preceptee relationship.

- Review patient handoffs and how the same concepts can be applied to preceptee handoffs.

- Discuss team communications.

- Role-play a difficult patient safety situation or handoff utilizing effective communication.

Chapter 7: Coaching

- Discuss coaching behaviors and beliefs.

- Discuss how to set up a coaching agreement. Engage participants in developing potential mutual agreements.

- Review the four-step coaching process.

- Use one or more case studies and have participants role-play coaching preceptees.

- Discuss resistance and edges. Use examples and/or case studies to have participants practice working with preceptee edges. Have participants use the four edge questions to role-play moving a preceptee or colleague through an edge or challenge.

- Discuss ending a preceptor-preceptee coaching relationship.

Chapter 8: Effectively Using Instructional Technologies

- Review the concept of E-learning and discuss examples of E-learning. If E-learning is used in your organization, allow preceptors to become familiar with any programs that their preceptees might use.

- Review web-based collaboration tools. Demonstrate wikis, blogs/vlogs, and podcasts.

- Discuss the concepts of simulation. Compare simulation fidelity.

- Discuss the use of role-playing, games, standardized patients, and virtual reality.

- Discuss the use of high-fidelity patient simulation and how it can be used to teach skills competency, critical thinking, clinical reasoning, and judgment.

- If your organization has simulators, demonstrate them to participants and provide them with information on how the simulators will be used with their preceptees. Allow participants to experience simulation scenarios themselves.

- Role-play a simulated clinical experience with preceptors so they can put into practice and demonstrate the knowledge they have gained regarding how to be an effective preceptor, with the faculty acting as the preceptee.

- Have preceptors complete a self-efficacy tool prior to simulation and again after simulation to assess their competence, confidence, and readiness to perform in the role of the preceptor.

Chapter 9: Precepting Specific Learner Populations

- Discuss precepting pre-licensure nursing students. Review agreements and forms from schools of nursing that have clinical rotations in your organization. Review role responsibilities and any limitations to student practice in your organization.

- Discuss the need for transition to practice programs for new graduate nurses. If your organization has an organized transition to practice program, review all aspects of the program with participants. Discuss the role of preceptors in the program. If there is no program or only a minimally organized program, discuss transition to practice in more detail.

- Ask participants to remember when they were new graduate nurses. Discuss what helped them through that transition and what hindered them.

- Review scopes of practice for nursing and other health care professionals in your state. Perhaps bring in some other health care professionals to discuss the scope of their practice.

- Discuss clinical autonomy. Have participants break into small groups and discuss expected levels of autonomous practice in your organization and in various units. Be specific about what nurses can do autonomously and what they cannot.

- Discuss precepting experienced nurses, newly hired experienced nurses, experienced nurses moving into a new specialty or role, and re-entry nurses. Review available resources.

- Review considerations for precepting internationally educated nurses and the practice gaps that result from education and culture.

- Discuss the generations of nurses in the workplace. Use music, television shows, or movies as examples of generational differences.

- Discuss the values and strengths that each generation brings to the workplace and generational differences in learning styles.

Chapter 10: Assessing and Addressing Preceptee Behavior and Motivation

- Discuss Just Culture as a problem-solving framework. Give participants examples of preceptee errors and have them discuss how they would apply Just Culture to working with preceptees on the errors.

- Review the Dimensional Model of Behavior as a tool to influence behavior change. Have participants discuss behavior examples and how they would deal with them.

- Discuss motivation in the workplace.

- Discuss using influence and the five-step process described in the article.

Chapter 11: Pragmatics of Precepting

- Discuss organization and time management, how to organize the shift for the preceptee, helping the preceptee organize and prioritize the work that needs to be done, and how to give shift report.

- Discuss strategies for assuring appropriate patient care assignments.

- Break the class into small groups and ask group members to share how they currently organize shifts. A representative from each group can share a summary of how a shift can be organized.

- Discuss the scopes of practice for your state (for example: RN, MD, pharmacist, respiratory therapist, LVN, CNA), concentrating on who can delegate to whom and under what conditions. Use examples.

- Develop a scenario describing a situation in which the preceptee displays unacceptable behaviors. The scenario should have preceptor, preceptee, and observer roles. Ask the group to role-play the scenario. Ask the preceptor, preceptee, and observer for feedback.

- Ask the group to share experiences when a preceptor-preceptee relationship did not work and how it was managed.

Chapter 12: For Managers: Selecting, Supporting, and Sustaining Preceptors

- Though this chapter is written for managers, the information can still be used in preceptor education.

- Review performance standards for preceptors if not done earlier in the course.

- Discuss with the group what successful outcomes would be with various preceptees (for example, new hires, new graduate nurses, clinical advancement for experienced nurses, etc.).

- Discuss how managers and preceptors can work together to assure that the preceptee is successful and safe.

- Discuss what would be meaningful recognition for the participants in their role as preceptor.

Chapter 13: The Practice of Self-Care to Prevent Burnout and Create the Optimal Healing Environment

- Discuss compassion fatigue and its effects on nurses.

- Discuss the concept of self-care. Break into small groups. Have participants review the pathway suggestions, select the ones that each of them wants to do, and discuss how they can support each other.

Index

A

AACN (American Association of Colleges of Nursing), 9, 76
AACN (American Association of Critical-Care Nurses), 136, 214
ABCD rule for developing objectives, 93
abstract conceptualization, 29
abstract random learning style, 27
abstract sequential learning style, 27
active experimentation, 29
adult learning. *See* learning, adult
Advanced Cardiac Life Support, 136
advocacy dialogue skill, 106–107, 111
affective domain, 79–80, 83
AHRQ (Agency for Healthcare Research and Quality), 5
Alfaro-LeFavre, 59, 63–64
American Heart Association, 136
American Philosophical Association, 60–62
ANA (American Nurses Association)
    Code of Ethics for Nurses, 4, 80, 214
    competence, position statement, 56
    competency, definition, 55–56
    Principles of Delegation, 204–206
    Standards of Nursing Practice, 3, 214
andragogy in practice model, 19

AORN (Association of periOperative Registered Nurses), 114, 169, 214
assignments, patient care, 200, 208–209
assistants, delegation to, 204–205
attitudes *vs.* behaviors, 178
autonomy, 167–168

B

Basic Life Support/Advanced Cardiac Life Support, 136
Bastable and Doody, 77, 79–81, 84, 90–91, 93, 95
behavioral objectives
    advantages, 90
    disadvantages, 90–91
Behavioral Pyramid
    Dimensional Model of Behavior and, 189
    influencing changes, 189–190
behaviors
    assessment of, 178–181, 187
    Behavioral Pyramid
        Dimensional Model of Behavior and, 189
        influencing changes, 189–190
    challenging, 210
    changes in, 187
    difficult conversations about, 115, 193–194
    Dimensional Model of Behavior, 182–190
        Behavioral Pyramid and, 189

people dimension, 183–184
quadrants of behavior patterns, 184–186
task dimension, 182–183
tips for using, 187
feedback about, 182, 186, 190
Five Step Format for influencing changes, 190–195
   develop action plan, 194–195
   get preceptee's views, 192–193
   give preceptor's views, 193–194
   resolve differences, 194
   start conversation, 191–192
fundamental attribution error, 179
group, 116
Just Culture framework, 179–181
   at-risk behavior, 180
   coaching and, 180–181
   external factors, 181
   human error, 179
   reckless behavior, 180
link to patient outcomes, 178
modeling, 20–21
motivation for, 188–190
observing, 20–21
resources for teaching, 252
vs. attitudes, 178
worksheet, 198, 212
Benner, Patricia, 23–24, 165–166, 218, 227
Blanchard, Ken *(The One Minute Manager)*, 44–45
Blink (Malcolm Gladwell), 67
blogs, 86, 138
Bloom's taxonomy
   affective domain, 79–80, 83
   Bloom's Digital Taxonomy, 84, 86
   Bloom's Original Taxonomy, 79–82
   cognitive domain, 79, 80, 83
   definition, 79
   evaluation, 81
   higher order thinking skills (HOTS), 81–82, 84–85

   knowledge dimension, 83
   lower order thinking skills (LOTS), 81–82, 84–85
   psychomotor domain, 80–81, 83–84
   Revised Bloom's Taxonomy, 81–84
   verb examples for domains, 83, 85–86
Bracey, 41

C

Churches, Andrew, 79–82, 84–86
clinical competence. *See* competency
clinical judgment
   definition, 65–66
   high-fidelity patient simulation and, 143
   model, 66
   Performance Based Development System (PBDS), 66–67, 165
   resources for teaching, 248
   worksheet, 73
clinical reasoning
   definition, 64
   deliberative rationality, 68–69
   developing, 67–69
   expert nurses, 38, 65, 68–69
   high-fidelity patient simulation and, 144
   intuition, 65, 67, 105
   patterns, 64–65
   rational choice strategy, 68
   recognition-primed decision model, 68
   resources for teaching, 248
   two systems, 65
   worksheet, 72
clinical teaching
   five minute preceptor model, 46–47
   microskills model, 45–46
   one-minute preceptor model, 44–47
   strengths-based approach, 43–44, 129

coaching
    4 Gateways Coaching
        address issue, 124–125, 127–128
        case study, 126–129
        clarify issue and outcome, 124–126
        identify actions and support, 124–126,
          128–129
        integrate learning, 124–126, 128
        questions to ask preceptee, 124–126
        Sample Coaching Worksheet, 125–126
    agreement with preceptee, 122–123
    behaviors and beliefs, 121–122
    edges, 130–131
    ending relationship with preceptee, 49–50,
      132
    guidelines for peer coaching, 129
    interaction formats, 124–130
    Just Culture framework and, 180–181
    preceptor's role, 121–133
    resistance, 130–131
    resources for teaching, 250
    strategies, 129–130
        appreciative inquiry, 108–109, 130
        strengths-based approach, 43–44, 129
    worksheet, 134
Code of Ethics for Nurses (ANA), 4, 80, 214
cognitive domain, 79, 80, 83
cognitive learning, 19, 26–28
communication
    advocacy dialogue skill, 106–107, 111
    delegation and, 205
    Dialogue Behaviors for Self checklist, 111
    dialogue beliefs, 104
    difficult conversations, 115, 193–194
    e-mail tips, 112
    groups
        "Full and Empty," poem on meetings,
          117
        behaviors in, 116
        check-in process, 116, 118

inquiry dialogue skill, 107, 111
    appreciative inquiry, 108–109, 130
    coaching questions, 108
    traditional process, 109
intent dialogue skill, 105, 111
ladder of inference, 106–107
listening dialogue skill, 105–106, 111
managing preceptors, 223–224
methods, managing, 112
patient handoffs
    AORN checklist, 114
    barriers to, 39
    ISBAR format, 113
    strategies for effective, 40
patient safety and, 112–113
resources for teaching, 249
self-improvement of dialogue skills, 111
sharing information, 39–40
silence dialogue skill, 110–111
teams and, 114–115
when to use dialogue skills, 104
competency
    characteristics, 59
    clinicians, 5
    Competency Outcomes and Performance
      Assessment (COPA), 57–58
    conscious competence model, 57
    definition (ANA), 55–56
    development, 58–59
    E-learning and, 137
    high-fidelity patient simulation and, 143
    newly competent nurses, 38
    performance discrepancies and, 207
    position statement (ANA), 56
    preceptor, 2
    professional, 2
    Quality and Safety Education for Nurses
      (QSEN), 5–6
    resources for teaching, 248
    safe medication administration and, 137
    worksheet, 72–73

Competency Outcomes and Performance Assessment (COPA), 57–58

concrete experience, 29

concrete random learning style, 27

concrete sequential learning style, 27

confidence (self-efficacy), 69, 248

conscious competence model, 57

context, of precepting, 2–8

continuum of fidelity, 140

continuums of learning, 29

converging learning style, 29

critical thinking
analysis, 61
characteristics of, 60–63
evaluation, 61
explanation, 61
inference, 61
interpretation, 61
nursing and, 62–63
precepting and, 63–64
resources for teaching, 61
self-regulation, 61
skills and sub-skills, 61
vs. thinking, 59
worksheet, 72

Crossing the Quality Chasm: A New Health System for the 21st Century (IOM), 4–5

Crucial Conversations: Tools for Talking When Stakes Are High, 115

culture
differences, internationally educated nurses, 171
norms, 149

cup colors teaching technique (Early), 42

CURE scale for prioritization, 201

Curry's classification system, 26

D

daily organization sheet, sample, 202

Daly, 123, 125, 130, 132

debriefing, 47–49, 147

delegation
assistants and, 204–205
communication and, 205
definition, 203
Five Rights of Delegation, 205
organizational accountability, 205–206
Principles of Delegation (ANA), 204–206
process (NCSBN), 203

deliberative rationality, 68–69

Dewey, John, 10, 49

dialogue. *See* communication

Dimensional Model of Behavior
Behavioral Pyramid and, 189
people dimension, 183–184
quadrants of behavior patterns, 184–186
task dimension, 182–183
tips for using, 187

diverging learning style, 29

documentation, 40, 170, 201–202, 223–224

domains of learning (Bloom), 79–81

Dossey, Barbara, 234

Doyle, Thomas, 140–141, 143

Dunn and Dunn, 30

E

E-learning
AACN online learning, 136
competencies and, 137
definition, 135–136
eDose program, 137
life support simulation, American Heart Association, 136
precepting and, 139

safe practice and, 137
Web-based collaboration, 137–139
    blogs/vlogs, 86, 138
    effectiveness of, 138–139
    podcasts, 138
    wikis, 138
Early, Sean, 42
edges (coaching), 130–131
eDose program, 137
education, nursing
    5-7, 141, 153, 165, 222, 116,168
ENA (Emergency Nurses Association), 214
environmental fidelity, 139–140
environmental issues, 39
equipment fidelity, 139–140
equipment issues, 39
Essentials of Critical Care Orientation (AACN),
    136
ethics, 2, 4, 80, 148–149, 214, 245
evaluation
    Bloom's taxonomy and, 81–83, 85–86
    critical thinking skills, 61
    guidelines for preceptor experience,
        161–162
    managing preceptors and, 225–227
    preceptee, 11, 152
evaluator (preceptor role), 11
evidence-based practice, 3, 5–6, 154
experienced nurses
    change specialties, 170
    clinical reasoning and, 65
    new to organization, 170
    preceptor roles and, 36
    programs for, 169
    re-entry into practice, 169
    resources for teaching, 251
    worksheet, 176
experiential learning, 10, 19, 23, 28–29, 47
expert nurses, 38, 68–69
extroversion-introversion dimension (Myers-
    Briggs), 27

F

facilitator (preceptor role), 10
Facione and Facione, 60–62, 65
feedback
    behaviors and, 182, 186, 190
    evaluator, 11
    five minute preceptor model, 46–47
    managing preceptors and, 225, 227
    preceptor-preceptee relationships and, 209
fidelity. *See also* high-fidelity patient
    simulation (HFPS)
    continuum of, 140
    environmental, 139–140
    equipment, 139–140
    psychological, 140
field dependence/independence, 28
Fink's taxonomy of significant learning
    application, 87–88
    caring, 87–89
    foundational knowledge, 87–88
    human dimension, 87–89
    implications for precepting, 88–90
    integration, 87–89
    learning how to learn, 87–90
    thinking, three types, 89
five minute preceptor model, 46–47
Five Rights of Delegation, 205
Five Step Format for influencing changes
    develop action plan, 194–195
    get preceptee's views, 192–193
    give preceptor's views, 193–194
    resolve differences, 194
    start conversation, 191–192
Four Gateways Coaching
    address issue, 124–125, 127–128
    case study, 126–129
    clarify issue and outcome, 124–126
    identify actions and support, 124–126,
        128–129
    integrate learning, 124–126, 128

questions to ask preceptee, 124–126
    sample coaching worksheet, 125–126
fundamental attribution error, 179
future of nursing initiative, 6–8

G

games, simulation, 140–141
gateways coaching. *See* coaching
Generation X, 171–173
Generation Y, 171–173
generations, precepting different
    Generation X, 171–173
    Generation Y/Millennials/Net
        Generation, 153, 171–173
    learning styles, 173
    resources for teaching, 251
    worksheet, 176
Gladwell, Malcolm *(Blink)*, 67
goals. *See also* taxonomies
    definition, 77
    interrelationship with objectives and
        outcomes, 77–78
    preceptor-preceptee relationships and, 208
    resources for teaching
    worksheet, 100–101
Grand Canyon University guidelines, 160–162
Gregorc's learning styles, 27
ground rules, 41–42
guidelines for formal meetings, 223–224

H

*Health Professions Education: A Bridge to
    Quality* (IOM), 5
hierarchy of learning pyramid (METI),
    144–145

hierarchy of needs (Maslow's)
    eight levels, 22
    five levels, 21
high-fidelity patient simulation (HFPS)
    adaptation, 151
    advantages, 143
    briefing, 146
    clinical competence and, 143
    clinical judgment and, 143
    clinical reasoning and, 144
    debriefing and, 147
    design, 145–147
    educator roles, 150–151
    ethics and, 148–149
    facilitation, 150–151
    foundational knowledge assurance, 146
    Jeffries model, 145
    knowledge development and, 149–150
    manager roles, 152
    patient safety and, 143–145
    practice, 146–147
    preceptor roles, 148–150
    quality improvement, 152
    reflective practice and, 147
    situation awareness, 144
higher order thinking skills (HOTS), 81–82,
    84–85
horizontal violence, 12–13
human behavior. *See* behaviors

I

influence without authority model, 9
information processing learning style, 28–29
inquiry dialogue skill, 107–109, 111
    appreciative inquiry, 108–109, 130
    coaching questions, 108
    traditional process, 109
instructional preferences learning style, 30

intent dialogue skill, 105, 111
internationally educated nurses
    practice gaps, 171
    resources for teaching, 251
    worksheet, 176
intuition, 65, 67, 105
IOM (Institute of Medicine), 4–8, 113

J

Jeffries model, high-fidelity patient simulation, 145
Johns model, reflective practice, 49
Johnson, Spencer *(The One Minute Manager)*, 44–45
judgment. *See* clinical judgment
judgment-perception dimension (Myers-Briggs), 27
Just Culture framework
    at-risk behavior, 180
    coaching and, 180–181
    external factors, 181
    human error, 179
    reckless behavior, 180

K

Keeping Patients Safe: Transforming the Work Environment of Nurses (IOM), 5
Klein, Gary, 67–68
knowledge of learner, prior, 19
Knowles, Malcolm, 17–20
Kolb, 28–29, 47
Kramer *(Reality Shock)*, 12

L

lateral violence, 12–13
leader/influencer (preceptor role), 9–10
learning continuums, 29
learning cycle, 29
learning styles
    abstract conceptualization, 29
    abstract random, 29
    accommodating, 29
    assimilating, 29
    characteristics of, 26
    cognitive, 26–28
    concrete random, 29
    concrete sequential, 29
    converging, 29
    Curry's classification system, 26
    diverging, 29
    experiential, 10, 19, 23, 28–29, 47
    field dependence/independence, 28
    Gregorc's, 27
    information processing, 28–29
    instructional preferences, 30
    Myers-Briggs Type Indicator (MTBI), 27
    resources for teaching
    sensory, 30
    worksheet, 33
learning taxonomies. *See* taxonomies
learning theories
    social, 20–21
    transformative, 20–21
learning theory, social, 20–21
learning theory, transformative, 20
learning, adult. *See also* taxonomies
    andragogy in practice model, 19
    assumptions about, 18
    individual differences, 19
    Knowles, Malcolm, 17–19
    principles of, 18
    progressing from simple to complex, 76

learning, experiential, 10, 19, 23, 28–29, 47

learning, facilitation of, 24

learning, Maslow's hierarchy of needs theory
  eight levels, 22
  five levels, 21

learning, novice to expert model, 23–25, 165–166, 218–219, 227

learning, resources for teaching, 246

Legacy Health
  Nursing Preceptor Rubric, 218
  Preceptor Evaluation, 226
  Preceptor Standards of Performance Development Model, 215
  Preferred Employee Profile, 217

Lenburg, 57–58

listening dialogue skill, 105–106, 111

lower order thinking skills (LOTS), 81–82, 84–85

Lucile Packard Children's Hospital, 170

M

Mager and Pipe, 206–207

managing preceptors
  challenges, 229
  communication and, 223–224
  educational opportunities, 222
  evaluation, 225–227
  feedback, 225, 227
  guidelines for formal meetings, 223–224
  Legacy Health Preceptor Evaluation, 225, 227
  match with preceptees
    conflicts, 221–222
    planning, 220
  mentorship programs, 229
  performance standards
    defining successful outcomes, 215
    Legacy Health model, 215
    organizational, 215

  professional organizations, 214–215
  unit-specific, 215

recognition
  examples, 228
  forms of, 228
  role of, 227

resources for teaching, 253

selection criteria
  Legacy Health Nursing Preceptor Rubric, 218
  Legacy Health Preferred Employee Profile, 216–217
  organization values and unit needs, 216

time management strategies, 229–230

worksheet, 231

Maslow's hierarchy of needs theory, 21–22
  eight levels, 22
  five levels, 21

METI, 144–145

microskills model, 45–46

Millennials, 171–173

modeling behavior, 20–21

models
  andragogy in practice, 19
  clinical judgment, 66
  Competency Outcomes and Performance Assessment (COPA), 57–58
  conscious competence, 57
  Dimensional Model of Behavior, 182–190
  five minute preceptor, 46–47
  influence without authority, 9
  Jeffries (HFPS), 145
  Johns (reflective practice), 49
  Legacy Health Preceptor Standards of Performance Development Model, 215
  microskills, 45–46
  novice to expert, 23–25, 165–166, 218–219, 227
  one-minute preceptor, 44–47
  precepting, 2
  preceptorship
    cohort of preceptees, 38–39

single preceptee, 38
single preceptor, 37
team preceptor, 37–38
rational choice strategy, 68
recognition-primed decision, 68
strengths-based approach, 43–44, 129
Transition to Practice (NCSBN), 165
trust-building, 41
motivation for behaviors, 188–190, 252
Mrs. Chase, 141
Myers-Briggs Type Indicator (MBTI), 27

N

NCSBN (National Council of State Boards of Nursing), 58–59, 163, 165, 203
Net Generation, 171–173
new graduate nurses
autonomy, 167–168
caring behavior of preceptors, 166–167
chaos of nursing unit, 167
life changes, 164
practice-education gap, 165
pre-licensure education, 168
resources for teaching, 251
scope of practice, 167
second-degree students, 169
transition to practice, 200–201
model (NCSBN), 165
residency programs, 7, 37–38, 165–166
new to organization, 170
newly competent nurses as preceptors, 38
NNSDO (National Nursing Staff Development Organization), 76, 169
novice to expert model, 23–25, 165–166, 218–219, 227
Nursing Preceptor Rubric (Legacy Health), 218
nursing, definition, 2

O

objectives. *See also* taxonomies
behavioral
advantages, 90
disadvantages, 90–91
cautions in developing, 95–96
elements of, 93
flexibility in planning, 76
interrelationship with goals and outcomes, 77–78
measurable, development of, 93–95
ABCD rule, 93
SMART rule, 94
resources for teaching, 249
verbs, examples of, 95
vs. outcomes, 76–78, 92
worksheet, 100–101
observing behavior, 20–21
one-minute preceptor model, 44–47
ONS (Oncology Nursing Society), 214
organization strategies
patient care assignments, 200, 208–209
preparing for shift, 200
prioritization, CURE scale, 201
resources for teaching, 252
sample daily organization sheet, 202
shift report, 200
transition to practice, 200–201
model (NCSBN), 165
residency programs, 7, 37–38, 165–166
worksheet, 212
organizational accountability, 205–206
orientation to job, 136, 166, 170, 223–224, 229
outcomes. *See also* taxonomies
definition (AACN), 76
development of desired, 76
expected of preceptee and preceptor, 35–36
interrelationship with objectives and goals, 77–78

measurable, development of, 93–94
    MATURE process, 94
    SMART rule, 94
resources for teaching, 249
statements, 91–92, 97
vs. objectives, 76–78, 92
worksheet, 100–101

P

patient care assignments, 200, 208–209, 252
patient handoffs
    AORN checklist, 114
    barriers to, 39
    ISBAR format, 113
    strategies for effective, 40
patient safety
    communication and, 112–113
    high-fidelity patient stimulation and,
      143–145
Performance Based Development System
  (PBDS), 66–67, 165
performance discrepancies
    check consequences, 207
    describe problem, 206
    develop solutions, 207
    enhance competence, 207
    explore fast fixes, 206
    implement solutions and reassess, 207–208
performance standards, managing
    defining successful outcomes, 215
    Legacy Health model, 215
    organizational, 215
    professional organizations, 214–215
    unit-specific, 215
podcasts, 138
poem on meetings, "Full and Empty," 117
positive clinical learning environment, 163–164
practice gaps, internationally educated nurses,
  171

practice-education gap, 165
pragmatics of precepting worksheet, 212
preceptee roles, 36, 41
preceptee-preceptor relationships. *See*
  preceptor-preceptee relationships
precepting model, 2
precepting strategies
    clinical teaching
      five minute preceptor model, 46–47
      microskills model, 45–46
      one-minute preceptor model, 44–47
      strengths-based approach, 43–44, 129
    debriefing, 47–49, 147
    E-learning and, 139
    ground rules, 41–42
    models of preceptorship
      cohort of preceptees, 38–39
      single preceptee, 38
      single preceptor, 37
      team preceptor, 37–38
    newly competent nurses as preceptors, 38
    patient handoffs
      AORN checklist, 114
      barriers to, 39
      ISBAR format, 113
      strategies for effective, 40
preceptee learner assessment, 42
preceptor-preceptee relationships, 208
    clinical goals, 208
    ending, 49–50, 132
    establishing, 41–42
    feedback and, 209
    manager's role in
      conflicts, 221–222
      planning, 220
    mismatch, 210–211
    patient care assignments, 200, 208–209
    resources for teaching, 252
    skill development, 208
reflective practice and, 49
resources for teaching, 247–248
role clarification, 35–36, 52–54

sharing information, 39–40
transitions into nursing, new role, new
    organization, 42–43
trust-building model, 41
worksheet, 52–53
precepting, definition, 1
Preceptor Evaluation (Legacy Health), 226
preceptor roles
    clarification of, 35–36, 41
    coaching and, 121–133
    evaluator, 11
    facilitator, 10
    Grand Canyon University guidelines, 161
    high-fidelity patient simulation and, 148–
        150
    leader/influencer, 9–10
    priority of, 35–36
    protector, 12–13
    resources for teaching, 245–246
    role model, 13
    socialization agent, 12
    teacher/coach, 8
    worksheet, 15
Preceptor Standards of Performance
    Development Model (Legacy Health), 215
preceptor-preceptee relationships
    clinical goals, 208
    ending, 49–50, 132
    establishing, 41–42
    feedback and, 209
    manager's role in
        conflicts, 221–222
        planning, 220
    mismatch, 210–211
    patient care assignments, 200, 208–209
    resources for teaching, 252
    skill development, 208
preceptorship models
    cohort of preceptees, 38–39
    single preceptee, 38
    single preceptor, 37
    team preceptor, 37–38

Preferred Employee Profile (Legacy Health), 217
Principles of Delegation (ANA), 204–206
prioritization, CURE scale, 201
priority of preceptor role, 35–36
process, delegation (NCSBN), 203
protector (preceptor role), 12–13
psychological fidelity, 140
psychomotor domain, 80–81, 83–84

Q

Quality and Safety Education for Nurses
    (QSEN), 5–6, 165
quality improvement, 6, 152
quality of care, 2, 5–6

R

rational choice strategy model, 68
re-entry into practice, 169
Reality Shock (Kramer), 12
reasoning. *See* clinical reasoning
recognition of preceptors
    examples, 228
    forms of, 228
    role of, 227
recognition-primed decision model, 68
recruitment strategies, 164
reflective observation, 29
reflective practice
    definition, 49
    Johns model, 49
    simulation and, 147
    strategies and, 49
relationships, preceptor-preceptee. *See*
    preceptor-preceptee relationships
residency programs, 7, 37–38, 165–166

resistance (coaching), 130–131

rewards, 45

role model (preceptor role), 13

roles of preceptor. *See* preceptor roles

Rudolph, 48–49

RWJF (Robert Wood Johnson Foundation), 5–7

S

safe learning environment, 12

safety education for nurses, 2, 5–6

safety, patient

    communication and, 112–113

    high-fidelity patient stimulation and, 143–145

scope of practice, 167, 252

selection criteria, for preceptors

    Legacy Health Nursing Preceptor Rubric, 218

    Legacy Health Preferred Employee Profile, 216–217

    organization values and unit needs, 216

self-care

    choices, 240–242

    choices pathway suggestions, 241–242

    compassion fatigue, 234

    definition, 234

    emotional, 237–238

    emotional pathway suggestions, 237–238

    mental, 235–237

    mental pathway suggestions, 236–237

    need for, 233–234

    physical, 234–235

    physical pathway suggestions, 235

    relationships, 239–240

    relationships pathway suggestions, 240

    resources for teaching, 252

    spiritual, 239

    spiritual pathway suggestions, 239

    Theory of Integral Nursing (Dossey), 234

    worksheet, 243

self-efficacy (confidence), 69, 248

sensing-intuitive dimension (Myers-Briggs), 27

sensory learning styles, 30

shift report, 200

silence dialogue skill, 110–111

simulation

    computer-assisted instruction, 140–141

    continuum of fidelity, 140

    environmental fidelity, 139–140

    equipment fidelity, 139–140

    games, 140–141

    hierarchy of learning pyramid (METI), 144–145

    high-fidelity patient simulation (HFPS)

        adaptation, 151

        advantages, 143

        briefing, 146

        clinical competence and, 143

        clinical judgment and, 143

        clinical reasoning and, 144

        debriefing and, 147

        design, 145–147

        educator roles, 150–151

        ethics and, 148–149

        facilitation, 150–151

        foundational knowledge assurance, 146

        Jeffries model, 145

        knowledge development and, 149–150

        manager roles, 152

        patient safety and, 143–145

        practice, 146–147

        preceptor roles, 148–150

        quality improvement, 152

        reflective practice and, 147

        situation awareness, 144

    history, 139

    integrated simulators, 140, 142

    METI, 144–145

    Mrs. Chase, 141

partial and complex task trainers, 140–141
psychological fidelity, 140
role-play, 140–141
standardized patients, 140–141
virtual reality and haptic-based systems,
  140–142
skill development, 208
SMART rule for developing objectives and
  outcomes, 94
social learning theory, 20–21
socialization agent (preceptor role), 12
specialties, changing, 170
staff involvement in precepting, 40
standardization, 39–40
Standards of Nursing Practice, ANA, 3–4
strategies, precepting. *See* precepting strategies
strengths-based approach, 43–44, 129
student nurses, 46, 159, 163–164
  agency responsibilities, 160–161
  college of nursing responsibilities, 160
  faculty advisor responsibilities, 162
  Grand Canyon University guidelines,
    160–162
  resources for teaching, 251
  student responsibilities, 162
support for preceptor/preceptee, 35–36

T

Tanner, Christine, 64–66, 143
taxonomies
  Bloom's taxonomy
    affective domain, 79–80, 83
    Bloom's Digital Taxonomy, 84, 86
    Bloom's Original Taxonomy, 79–82
    cognitive domain, 79, 80, 83
    definition, 79
    evaluation, 81
    higher order thinking skills (HOTS),
      81–82, 84–85
    knowledge dimension, 83
    lower order thinking skills (LOTS),
      81–82, 84–85
    psychomotor domain, 80–81, 83–84
    Revised Bloom's Taxonomy, 81–84
    verb examples for domains, 83, 85–86
  Fink's taxonomy of significant learning
    application, 87–88
    caring, 87–89
    foundational knowledge, 87–88
    human dimension, 87–89
    implications for precepting, 88–90
    integration, 87–89
    learning how to learn, 87–90
    thinking, three types, 89
  scaffolding learning, 81, 137
teacher/coach (preceptor role), 8
teaching. *See* clinical teaching
technology, instructional. *See also* E-learning;
  simulation
    future of, 154–155
      privacy concerns, 154–155
      smartphones, 154
    Net Generation and
      characteristics, 153
      educational needs, 153
    resources for teaching, 250
    worksheet, 157
*The Future of Nursing: Leading Change,
  Advocating Health* (IOM), 6–8
The Joint Commission, 113
The One Minute Manager, 44–45
Theory of Integral Nursing, 234
thin-slicing of experience, 67
thinking-feeling dimension (Myers-Briggs), 27
time for precepting, 35–36, 39
time management
  patient care assignments, 200, 208–209
  preparing for shift, 200
  prioritization, CURE scale, 201
  resources for teaching, 252
  sample daily organization sheet, 202

shift report, 200
transition to practice, 200–201
    model (NCSBN), 165
    residency programs, 7, 37–38, 165–166
worksheet, 212
To Err Is Human: Building a Safer Health System
  (IOM), 4
transformative learning theory, 20
transition to practice, 165–166, 200–201
    model (NCSBN), 165
    residency programs, 7, 37–38, 165–166
transitions into nursing, new role, new
  organization, 42–43
trust-building model, 41

V

values, 9–10
values conflicts, 10
verbs
    examples for Bloom's taxonomy domains,
      83, 85–86
    examples for objectives, 95
Versant RN residency, 37–38
vlogs, 138

W

Web-based collaboration
    blogs/vlogs, 86, 138
    effectiveness of, 138–139
    podcasts, 138
    wikis, 138
Wesorick and Shiparski, 104–106, 108, 110
Wikipedia, 138
wikis, 138
worksheet, 176